Carte Blanche
The Erosion
of Medical Consent

COLUMBIA GLOBAL REPORTS
NEW YORK

Carte Blanche
The Erosion of
Medical Consent

Harriet A. Washington

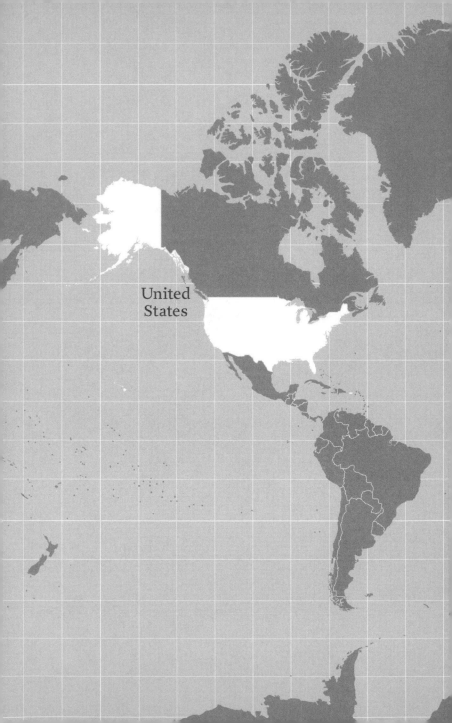

United
States

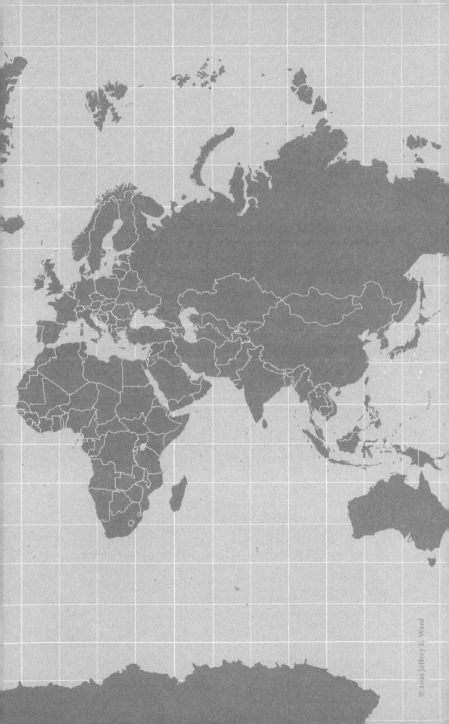

For Ron DeBose

Support for this book was provided in part by the Robert Wood Johnson Foundation. The views expressed here do not necessarily reflect the views of the Foundation.

Carte Blanche:
The Erosion of Medical Consent

Published by Columbia Global Reports
91 Claremont Avenue, Suite 515
New York, NY 10027
globalreports.columbia.edu
facebook.com/columbiaglobalreports
@columbiaGR

Library of Congress Cataloging-in-Publication Data
Names: Washington, Harriet A., author.
Title: Carte Blanche: The Erosion of Medical Consent / Harriet A. Washington.
Description: New York, NY : Columbia Global Reports, [2021] | Includes
    bibliographical references. |
Identifiers: LCCN 2020040295 (print) | LCCN 2020040296 (ebook) | ISBN
    9781734420722 (paperback) | ISBN 9781734420739 (ebook)
Subjects: MESH: Informed Consent--ethics | Human Experimentation--ethics |
    Researcher-Subject Relations--ethics | United States
Classification: LCC R853.H8 (print) | LCC R853.H8 (ebook) | NLM W 20.55.H9 | DDC
    174.2/8--dc23
LC record available at https://lccn.loc.gov/2020040295
LC ebook record available at https://lccn.loc.gov/2020040296

Book design by Strick&Williams
Map design by Jeffrey L. Ward
Author photograph by Aaron Mayes, University of Nevada at Las Vegas (UNLV)

Printed in the United States of America

CONTENTS

Informed Consent in the Time of Infection

It was mid-May in 2020 when Robin Armstrong declared victory over the coronavirus.

Armstrong, a doctor at a nursing home called The Resort in Texas City, described giving the anti-malarial drug hydroxychloroquine to dozens of nursing home employees and patients in his care who suffered from COVID-19. Armstrong told reporters that hydroxychloroquine demonstrated its safety and effectiveness when thirty-five of his patients recovered and only three died. However, he produced no documentation to support this claim, and the Galveston County Health District has not verified it. In fact, county health officials say retesting of forty infected patients at The Resort found that nineteen still tested positive, and that there were five new cases.

Armstrong admitted having given the drug to scores of elderly patients, some of whom suffered from dementia, making them unable to offer informed consent. Armstrong also failed to elicit consent from the designated family members who could give consent in their stead.

Two months previously, U.S. president Donald Trump had begun touting hydroxychloroquine on Twitter. By April, vice president Mike Pence announced that hydroxychloroquine was to be used in several drug trials covering, for example, three thousand patients at a hospital in Detroit. Pence told a White House briefing that they were "more than prepared" to make hydroxychloroquine available to doctors' offices and pharmacies in the Detroit area.

Without evidence, President Trump insisted that hydroxychloroquine be pressed into service as a treatment for coronavirus. In addition to the paucity of supporting data and Trump's lack of scientific acumen, his championing of the drug was marred by conflicts of interest, including his interest in European stock-market index funds and in French drugmaker Sanofi, which manufactures the medication.

From March 9 to 19, prescriptions for hydroxychloroquine spiked by 367 percent. The medication is approved for use against malaria and it is legal for U.S. physicians to prescribe FDA-approved medications for other, "off-label," uses. Moreover, the FDA specifically issued hydroxychloroquine an Emergency Use Authorization against COVID-19 in March. Still, prescribing must adhere to ethical requirements that include informing a patient or the patient's representative, in cases where the patient is incapable of giving or withholding consent. But were patients being informed of hydroxychloroquine's experimental nature and its risks? Did they have a chance to say *yes* or *no* to this experimental medication?

On April 23, Helen Edrozo died at the age of eighty-seven after Armstrong gave her hydroxychloroquine and her condition rapidly worsened. Edrozo's dementia precluded informed

10   consent and her son says he was not consulted. Larry Edrozo questions whether the drug might have hastened his mother's decline. Across the nation, nursing homes had barred family members to discourage the spread of infection, and The Resort was no exception, but Armstrong could have explained the medication regimen and arranged to obtain consent by telephone.

Armstrong was unapologetic about not having done so, telling *Houston Chronicle* reporters Nick Powell and Taylor Goldenstein, "If I had to call all the families for every medicine that I started on a patient, I wouldn't be treating any patients at all. I would just be talking to families all the time."

Armstrong's defense evokes the pressures of clinical urgency, a common plea for dispensing with consent that will be revisited often in this book. The staggeringly high rates of coronavirus infection in nursing homes filled with susceptible elderly certainly constitutes an emergency, but it does not present an excuse for abandoning ethical behavior, especially when caring for the powerless who cannot effectively express their own opinions about their medical fate nor advocate for themselves.

Although Trump's fondness for and financial interest in the drug led to its endorsement by many of his political followers, most medical experts soon took a much dimmer view of its appropriateness for coronavirus treatment. By mid-April, an effectiveness study of hydroxychloroquine's analogue chloroquine in Brazil was cut short when subjects developed irregular heartbeats and eleven people died within six days. The FDA revoked authorization for hydroxychloroquine coronavirus treatment on June 15, noting in part that "recent data from a large randomized controlled trial showed no evidence of benefit for mortality or other outcomes such as hospital length

of stay or need for mechanical ventilation of HCQ treatment in
hospitalized patients with COVID-19."

Armstrong serves as a Texas Republican national party
committee member and even nominated Trump for president at
the 2016 Republican National Convention. Conflicts of interest
entail social, professional, and political benefits as well as financial ones, and it is reasonable to ask whether Armstrong's political fealty influenced his medical judgment in this case.

Withholding Care

What precisely is informed consent? Most of us have a notion,
however vague, that in twenty-first-century America, patients
can't be coerced into medical research without their permission, and that this permission must be not only voluntary but
also informed by a useful knowledge of what the research entails.
Many people, and even some healthcare workers, consider
informed consent a piece of paper, a document signed by the subject to indicate her understanding of the study's purpose, requirements, and other pertinent details, including known risks.

But informed consent is much more than a piece of
paper. Informed consent helps to enforce ethical principles of
autonomy, beneficence, and justice, and the signed form is only
one piece of evidence buttressing a researcher's claim that she
has explained everything a subject reasonably needs to know in
order to make the best decision about whether he wants to participate. The researcher should impart information guided by
the question: What would the average patient need to know to
be an informed participant in the decision? She also should bear
in mind the question: What would a typical physician say about
this research study?

The subject must be provided information about the study's purpose, requirements, design, known risks, possible discomfort, and putative benefits. Subjects must be informed of all their options in addition to participating in the study, including the option to take an approved, tested treatment, to pursue nonpharmaceutical treatment instead, or to pursue no treatment at all. The exchange is confidential except that FDA staff may read it. The protocol, or blueprint for the medical research, must lay out and explain whether compensation or treatment will be provided for adverse events, and that the subject can leave the study at any time, whether she has been paid or not. Contact information must be provided for a staff person to consult, in case further questions arise.

Informed consent also means warning the subject about possible lifestyle effects. Will he be fatigued? Feel discomfort? Be unable to sleep, or to drive? Informed consent is continuous, not static, so any developments or discoveries that emerge throughout the study, such as adverse effects that might impinge upon a subject's decision to continue in the study, must be shared with the subjects. The responsibility to communicate this information persists throughout the study so that subjects must be warned about, for example, any dangerous effects that emerge during the study. And informed consent can manifest quite differently when a patient is considering treatment than when a subject is considering enrolling in research.

Imposing questionable drugs like hydroxychloroquine without informed consent is just one example of coronavirus-fueled consent evasion. The right to consent has also been abandoned by those who advocate *withholding* essential treatment. The scarcity of medical personnel, protective gear, and basic technology has led various institutions to limit or withhold treatment from some coronavirus patients without their permission or even their knowledge. Variously described as limiting, rationing, or triage, withholding care from those deemed to have a poor quality of life or those for whom treatment is assumed to be futile, the policies rob patients of their right to consent.

As hospitals, nursing homes, and prisons find it necessary to bar access by patients' families and other visitors, those institutions are transformed into closed systems. Thus, nonconsensual rationing takes place in secrecy, as families complain that treatment plans are obscured or withheld from them altogether.

One of the most chilling of these policies was adopted in Newark, New Jersey, where cardiopulmonary resuscitation, or CPR, for COVID-19 patients was withheld.

Once flashing lights and screaming sirens heralded the ambulance's arrival, Newark paramedics would rush to their victims, but if they found that the patient had "flatlined," meaning that there was no heartbeat, the EMTs did not work to save him. No cardiopulmonary resuscitation was begun. No epinephrine was injected in an attempt to restart the heart. No defibrillator was pulled out to shock the heart back into a normal rhythm. The sirens were silenced, the lights turned off, and no CPR was offered.

EMTs withheld CPR because they feared contracting coronavirus despite protective gear. So, in Newark and some other cities in New Jersey and New York, they declared these victims dead at the scene, without trying CPR or other elements of the standard of care. New York has since reversed its policy that banned CPR but municipalities in some states continued

14   to withheld CPR altogether; in Texas and Louisiana, EMTs reduced the average time that they administered CPR from forty minutes to about ten minutes.

The infectious-disease risk is real, but it is nothing new. Healthcare workers treat a plethora of infectious diseases, yet suspending lifesaving care has not been widely pondered since the early years of the HIV/AIDS pandemic sowed similar fear among healthcare workers. HIV was another novel and murkily understood infectious disease, and there's much we still don't understand about coronavirus transmission. The same fear of the unknown may have triggered the desire in the 1980s and 1990s to withhold care from the HIV-positive, a suggestion that was unethical in the past and is unethical now.

In both cases the discussions have taken place in venues— medical literature, conferences, and professional meetings— where the laypersons most affected by these dramatic and dangerous policy changes are absent and unconsulted.

Even more insidious are policies floated specifically to withhold care from the elderly and disabled on the basis that doctors deem them to contribute less to society, to have a poor quality of life, or both.

Not all these measures are confined to the disabled. Anyone infected with coronavirus can fall prey to other schemes to withhold care. For example, some institutions and hospitals ponder mandatory "do not resuscitate" orders (DNRs), that would limit the lifesaving care offered patients by denying treatment, food, and water—which would condemn COVID-19 patients to death. Unlike standard DNRs, this withholding or withdrawal of care would be imposed without the consent of the patient or her family and perhaps without her knowledge.

Such policies hearken back to an openly eugenic past.
For example, in 1915, Dr. Harry J. Haiselden allowed Anna
Bollinger's baby boy to die in the hospital because "he would
have gone through life as a defective." In the next three years
Haiselden killed five other babies by withholding care, and the
press covered the topic uncritically. Haiselden called for others
to follow his practice of negative eugenics by killing the "genetically inferior." He even starred in a successful feature film, *The
Black Stork,* which dramatized his eugenic message by glori-
fying the death of a genetically "tainted" child. Around the same
time, in Berlin's 4 Tiergartenstrasse offices, 230,000 people
with physical or mental disabilities were ordered murdered in
its "T4" program as "useless eaters" by physicians. Passively
withholding care from the disabled and actively administering
agents to cause their death seem very different steps, but history shows us that it is but a step from one act to the other.

Today, imposing mandatory DNR orders for coronavirus
patients is a shocking departure from normal DNR orders that
are imposed in order to maximize the patient's welfare and only
with the patient's full understanding and voluntary consent. For
example, studies have long shown that administering cardiac
resuscitation to most patients over the age of eighty-five has a
poor risk-benefit ratio. Such patients rarely leave the hospital
alive, but often suffer broken ribs and other injuries that tend
to result in a poorer state of health and quality of life than if the
resuscitation had not been undertaken. The caregiver explains
this to the patient and to his surrogate, health proxy, or family
member—who should be included in discussions even when the
patient retains decision-making capacity. Only after explaining
this and determining and recording the patient's goals for care

16   and treatment preferences will the patient's choice to accept or
reject DNR be made. Only if the patient agrees will a DNR stipulate which interventions will and will not be undertaken in an
emergency. If the patient insists he wants every possible medical attention taken, no DNR goes into effect.

But some newly instituted policies for coronavirus treatment mandate blanket DNRs for all with COVID-19 no matter
their clinical picture or their ability or willingness to accept or
withstand emergency interventions. In these cases, the nonconsensual DNR is imposed to ease the burden on the medical staff,
not to maximize the health of the patients. Moreover, patients,
their families, and their representatives are not informed of the
DNR and have no opportunity to reject it.

Denying Care

COVID-19 policies have also dealt with widespread shortages
of preventive gear, ventilators, ICU beds, and staff by adopting
policies that limit care to some through rationing. Perhaps the
most insidious form entails a species of triage in which institutions in a slew of states adopted policies that withheld access
to lifesaving ventilators not only from COVID-19 patients but
also from disabled people who have long depended upon the
technology to live. Alabama, Kansas, Tennessee, and Washington invoked the urgency of the pandemic and the scarcity of
machines to withdraw ventilators from the elderly and the disabled, even those who had long relied on the technology to live.
On March 23, advocates for the disabled complained to the U.S.
Department of Health and Human Services' Civil Rights Office
that rationing plans promulgated by the state of Washington
and the University of Washington Medical Center gave priority

"to treating people who are younger and healthier, and leaves those who are older and sicker—people with disabilities—to die."

In response, the HHS office issued a bulletin on March 28, reminding health providers that they could not discriminate as they provided treatment and care to patients afflicted by COVID-19. This warning did not stop the neoeugenic discussions, and seems not to have prevented the nonconsensual withholding of care.

Melissa Hickson says that her husband, Michael, a wheelchair-bound forty-six-year-old African American father of five with coronavirus, died on June 11 at Texas's South Austin Medical Center after medication, food, and water were withheld from him for six days in contravention to her stated wishes.

The doctor caring for him had told her that Hickson would no longer be treated because he was wheelchair-bound and had no "quality" of life.

But she disagrees. Michael Hickson, who had been left a quadriplegic after a heart attack in 2017, had "regained his personality, had memories of past events, loved to do math calculations, and answer trivia questions," she told the *Texan* in an article illustrated by a beaming Hickson surrounded by his five smiling children. She recalled a conversation with the attending physician:

> "So as of right now, his quality of life—he doesn't have much of one," the doctor said.
>
> "What do you mean? Because he's paralyzed with a brain injury, he doesn't have quality of life?" she responded
>
> "Correct," the doctor replied.

18   Withholding care by refusing to perform CPR and withdrawing care by ceasing to give medicine, food, and water may seem like very different medical actions, but most experts agree that they are ethically equivalent. The American Medical Assocation's *Code of Medical Ethics* notes that "while there may be an emotional difference between not initiating an intervention at all and discontinuing it later in the course of care, there is no ethical difference between withholding and withdrawing treatment . . . when an intervention no longer helps to achieve the patient's goals for care or desired quality of life, it is ethically appropriate for physicians to withdraw it." The U.S. courts have supported this. But in COVID-19 cases like Hickson's, it is not the patients' welfare and autonomy that determine whether care is offered or denied—it is the convenience and welfare of others.

The U.S. is not alone in this. On March 21, the United Kingdom's National Institute for Health and Care Excellence (NICE) indicated that patients should not receive ventilation if they were classified as "frail," according to a medical rating designed for the elderly but that includes people who have difficulty dressing or bathing themselves, as well as those with autism or learning disorders.

Consent Optional
Outrage greeted the proposals in April from French physicians Camille Locht, research director for France's National Institute of Health and Medical Research (Inserm), and Jean-Paul Mira, head of ICU services at the Cochin Hospital, concerning ethically questionable placebo studies, in which a large proportion of the subjects receive no treatment at all for a serious disorder.

Placebo studies for serious or fatal diseases are ethically unacceptable in the West because some in the study receive no
treatment for the disease but only a faux treatment, or placebo, popularly characterized as a "sugar pill." These may confer
poorly understood benefits via the "placebo effect," but such
effects are weak. Medications tend to outperform placebos.

So, in the West, research studies offer all subjects some
treatment, preferably the standard of care. But thanks to
changes in the Declaration of Helsinki that governs the conduct
of research in the developing world, it requires only standard
of care in the country where the research is conducted, and in
much of the Global South the standard of care is: nothing.

Placebo trials have come to be frowned upon in the West, so
Locht and Mira proposed that such trials be conducted in Africa
instead.

"A bit like it is done for some studies on AIDS, where with
prostitutes, we try things because we know that they are highly
exposed and they don't protect themselves," Mira added during
a conversation.

Mira's reference to "prostitutes . . . who do not protect
themselves" invokes a tacit assumption that Africans' "immo-
rality" makes them less worthy of the respect afforded white
subjects' lives. This disdain is revealed in the comparison to the
equally unethical use of women to test early HIV antiretrovirals,
some of whom were prostitutes, but many of whom were not.
Mira reveals the tendency to blame the victim, suggesting that
irresponsible Africans are responsible for their own diseases

"You are right," Camille Locht responded. "And we are in the
process of thinking about a study in Africa in parallel to carry
out the same type of approach with BCG, a placebo."

Pearl-clutching media coverage and public outrage was followed by the inevitable apologies. However, the doctors' question was not a novel one, but simply the conduct of unethical research as usual. As I discussed in the African journal *Mondafrique,* I had seen this very suggestion proposed and discussed in the medical literature for many years, sans outrage.

Four-fifths of corporate clinical trials are now conducted in the developing world where high-quality studies can be completed much more quickly and cheaply than in the United States. The Declaration of Helsinki that governs the conduct of trials abroad provides for lower standards of protection than does the U.S. Code of Federal Regulations, which governs U.S. research, and many cases of research without informed consent have resulted.

The proposal to use African patients to test medications thousands of miles from the millions of COVID-19 infections in the West is unethical for several reasons. Africans are being asked to assume all the risks of the research but are unlikely to benefit proportionately, if at all—both because there were far fewer cases in most African countries and also because once approved in African studies, branded Western medications typically are priced out of the reach of Africans. I remember, for example, that nearly everyone argued against making ZMapp available to Africans in the 2014 Ebola outbreak. It was withheld even from Sierra Leone's chief virologist, Dr. Sheik Umar Khan, who died of Ebola. I was one of the few ethicists to argue that Africans should receive the drug.

U.S. medical researchers must adhere to U.S. law but oversight is scarce. The U.S. relies on scientists' assurance that they have conducted research legally and ethically, but too often they have not¯as when Pfizer had to pay a settlement when children died and were injured during a study of the antibiotic Trovan conducted by U.S. researchers in the midst of a Nigerian meningitis epidemic. Informed consent forms "went missing" and a doctor admitted to forging the required hospital permission form after the fact. Moreover, Africa has harbored a number of high-profile Western medical miscreants who have intentionally administered deadly agents under the guise of providing healthcare or conducting research.

Yet public-health experts and the news media express frustration and wonder at the fears that may make African Americans loath to embrace novel treatments, including the several COVID-19 vaccine candidates whose manufacturer claimed more than 90 percent efficacy as this book went to press. When vaccines are deemed ready for market on the basis of truncated, expedited testing and claims of unsubstantiated by peer review, we should evaluate any reticence in a more objective manner. Instead of interrogating the fears of people of color and deploying labels like "anti-vaxxer" and "vaccine-hesitant," the better question is "How can we meaningfully improve the trustworthiness of the U.S. healthcare system, especially as it relates to reinforcing transparency and informed consent in COVID-19 vaccine research?"

Finally, infection itself can sabotage informed consent, necessitating greater care in establishing strategies to preserve patient and subject consent. In 2015, I documented infection as a neglected risk factor for both mental illness and cognitive

22   deterioration in my book *Infectious Madness: The Surprising Science of How We "Catch" Mental Illness* and my article "The Well Curve" in the *American Scholar*.

Influenza outbreaks, including the 1918–20 pandemic to which COVID-19 is so often compared, have been followed by waves of mental disease and cognition loss. These ailments include schizophrenia and neuropsychiatric symptoms including anxiety, depression, mania, memory loss, psychosis, and delirium. The Oliver Sacks book *Awakenings* about brain devastation in the influenza pandemic's aftermath brought wide awareness to this phenomenon when it was made into a feature film starring Robert De Niro and Robin Williams in 1990.

We've known since April that the COVID-19 survivors suffer neurological symptoms including the loss of hearing and taste, as well as encephalopathy that creates changes in consciousness. According to a report in *Brain, Behavior, and Immunity*, one in five known cases suffers delirium triggered by "cytokine storm syndrome."

It's too early to look for definitive data about the infection's long-term cognitive effects, but neurologic problems haunted 78 of 214 patients in a study of those who tested positive for COVID-19. Strokes, which cause cognitive losses of memory, speech, and intellectual functioning, also affect previously young and healthy COVID-19 survivors. A 2009 *Archives of Internal Medicine* study found that survivors of SARS-CoV-1 have been clinically diagnosed with PTSD (54.5 percent), depression (39 percent), pain disorder (36.4 percent), panic disorder (32.5 percent), and obsessive-compulsive disorder (15.6 percent) thirty-one to fifty months postinfection, a dramatic increase

from their preinfection prevalence of any psychiatric diagnoses
(3 percent).

Coronavirus leaves a lingering, and perhaps permanent, damage to the neurological system and to cognitive ability, which easily sabotages survivors' ability to give or withhold consent to medical procedures and to medical research. These lingering deficits may even fuel the regrettable tendency of some clinicians to question survivors' quality of life as an antecedent to withholding medical care.

Exigencies of War

A hospital alone shows what war is.
—Erich Maria Remarque

Private First Class Jemekia Barber, of the 7th Infantry Division, is the custodian of a proud military heritage. In 2003 she was twenty-three and stationed with her husband at Fort Carson, Colorado, and as I read *Jemekia Barber v. the United States of America*, her story evoked my own past.

My parents, a WAC (Women's Army Corps) soldier and a paratrooper, had also served in the Army, meeting and marrying at Fort Dix, New Jersey, where I was born. As we moved from base to base and country to country, the friendships and culture peculiar to Army life defined and enriched my early life in ways that only other military brats fully understand. For years after my parents left the military for traditional corporate life and homemaking, I was haunted by a sense of exile.

So, after reading Barber's legal briefs, I was braced for bitterness as I dialed her telephone number. As the daughter of two soldiers, I understand what it means to be cast out by the military when "the service" is a family tradition.

Barber accepted my out-of-the-blue phone call graciously and proceeded to coolly recite facts that portrayed a cruel game of soldier's roulette. Her pleasantly modulated voice hinted at no angst or ethical outrage, but her precise, clear account suppressed neither her wistfulness nor flashes of pride in her military heritage, a tradition she now can never share.

"My husband was in the military. My brother is still in the military. My grandfather was in World War II, and my uncle Joseph Neil Spelling served in the Marines. He died before I was born—a hero, while saving people's lives." Even her in-laws, both of them, saw service in Vietnam.

But she was driven from the Army in disgrace after being confined to the brig for refusing to obey orders, after which she fled. She went briefly AWOL. Then she sued the Army—and lost. She narrowly escaped a court-martial for her infractions, and was denied an honorable discharge.

Her crime? She refused to take a six-shot series of experimental anthrax vaccinations. The decision for *Barber v. United States Army* explains:

> While still in active service, Ms. Barber was ordered to receive an anthrax vaccination in preparation for a transfer to Korea. She disobeyed that order on the ground that the vaccination may not be safe for females of child-bearing age.

Barber doesn't deny this. "I have refused to submit to the injections because my own research led me to believe that submitting will lead to irreversible health problems or other serious adverse consequences." She explained to me, "We were taken to a hospital on post and given printouts saying that there were no adverse reactions and that the various drugs had been approved by the FDA in 1999 or January 2000. But a pregnant girl in my command had taken two anthrax shots and when she went to the doctor one day he said 'the baby is gone.' Having children was important to us but the warning labels suggest it may be harmful to fertility."

Her account suggests she was misled concerning the "approved" status of the vaccine. It was approved only for cutaneous anthrax affecting the skin, but not for the deadlier inhalation anthrax that soldiers faced. The vaccine was unapproved for this use and the U.S. Army hoped that data from the involuntary injections would establish its safety profile and effectiveness. In short, it was experimental.

The admonitions in the vaccine's product insert did nothing to quell concerns about the vaccine and pregnancy. The insert read in part, "Studies have not been performed to ascertain whether Anthrax Vaccine Adsorbed has carcinogenic action, or any effect on fertility."

"We did research and found other people who were disabled because of the shot. I didn't want to take the shot. I could not agree to that, because having children was important to us."

She recalls that another soldier, like her an African American, "had 20/20 vision before he took the shots: he lost 80 percent of the vision in one eye and 40 percent in the other eye. After the third shot, he feared he would die, but the Army says it was a reaction to Tylenol."

The trend toward overrepresentation of minority groups in nonconsensual research was borne out with the vaccination program. Soldiers of all races were affected by the compulsory anthrax vaccinations, but Blacks were overrepresented because they constituted 12.3 percent of Americans, but were 24.5 percent of the 1.7 million ground troops deployed to the Gulf in 1990 and 26.2 percent of Army reservists in 2001—twice their representation in the population at large, and so at twice the risk of being forced into military research.

Barber was far from alone in being commanded to undergo anthrax immunization: Safety concerns also caused Private Kamila Iwanowska of New York City to shun "the shot." She told her superiors she thought the shot could endanger her future children, adding that the vaccine's long-term effects were unknown. "The side effects I read about were alarming: There were a lot of people who were getting sick from that," she told CBS News. Upon her refusal, Iwanowska, then twenty-six, was court-martialed and given a bad-conduct discharge in 2003.

By October 2001, at least four hundred soldiers had been disciplined, including court-martials and jailing, for refusing the mandatory inoculation. Many personnel who received the shots complained of mysterious autoimmune symptoms and illnesses, although the Pentagon publicly insisted the vaccine was both effective and safe. It attributed complaints to "emotional issues"—even those reports made by military doctors and other health workers. The military subsumed vaccine-related illnesses under the nebulous symptomatology of "Gulf War Syndrome."

Lt. Col. Frank Fischer, MD, who was forced to take the vaccine while serving in the Air Force Reserve Medical Corps, says the health worker who administered the vaccine to him refused to answer his questions, and that he suffers autoimmune symptoms in the aftermath of the vaccination. Rich Rovet, an Air Force

28   nurse, testified before a congressional hearing about physical harms he saw and complained publicly that vaccine-damaged servicepeople were treated unconscionably without recourse.

Why had they no recourse? If they were injured as a result of being forced by an employer to take potentially harmful medication, especially an experimental one, most people would consider suing for damages. However, such a lawsuit is not an option for injured soldiers because of the Feres doctrine.

This version of sovereign immunity arose from a trio of unsuccessful 1950 suits brought by soldiers against the Army, called *Feres v. United States*. In one case, a thirty-inch towel bearing the logo "Medical Department U.S. Army" was found in the abdomen of a soldier undergoing an operation. His legal complaint alleged it was left by a negligent Army surgeon, a claim that could hardly be rebutted. But the judge barred him and all service members from holding the government liable for injures they receive in the course of service, even should the harms result from negligence.

This explains why, although other soldiers had been injured by the vaccine, Barber's was the first anthrax vaccination issue to go before a civilian court. Her lawyers asked federal courts for an injunction against the mandatory vaccinations on the grounds that they would threaten any pregnancy and represent an unconstitutional denial of her rights. Barber didn't make the decision to sue lightly, she explained to me. She had exhausted all her other options.

But why was the U.S. Department of Defense so adamant about forcing an experimental anthrax vaccine on all soldiers and reservists who saw active duty? Because U.S. combatants

were being deployed to lands where anthrax might pose a
threat—either naturally, because anthrax is endemic to much
of the world, or via weaponized warfare. Rumors abounded that
the CIA was itself stockpiling anthrax; however, the DOD feared
its use by our enemies—Iraq in the Gulf War, and elsewhere.
The DOD knew the existing vaccine was effective against skin
but not inhaled anthrax and it wanted to know as soon as possible whether it would afford enough protection to soldiers suffering inhalation exposure.

Since antiquity, we've known that anthrax is characterized by a constellation of flu-like symptoms, including muscle
aches, sore throat, mild fever, fatigue and shortness of breath,
chest pain, nausea, coughing up blood, and pain on swallowing.
But it is the purplish black chancres sprouting on the skin of
the infected that gave anthrax its name, from *xylánthrakas*, the
Greek word for charcoal.

Humans can become infected through direct or indirect
contact with infected livestock, game, and their body parts, so
historically, anthrax has been an occupational hazard for farm
and slaughterhouse workers. The disease is caused when the
spores of bacterium *Bacillus anthracis* enter the body through
breaks in the skin, abdominal wounds, injection, or most dangerously, through inhalation. Left untreated, inhalation anthrax
kills more than 90 percent of those infected. Even those treated
with antibiotics often succumb.

Throughout the nineteenth century, sporadic natural outbreaks struck animals and the humans who lived close to them.
But mystifying early twentieth-century outbreaks struck bar-
bers and soldiers, people with no apparent contact with infected

30   animals. Scientists learned that spore-contaminated horse hair used in shaving brushes was killing them quite effectively.

Many even credit anthrax with the death of Reinhard Heydrich, the notorious "Butcher of Prague" and chief architect of Hitler's murderous "final solution," which he planned at the 1942 Wannsee Conference in Berlin. On May 27 of that year, a small group of Czech patriots ambushed Heydrich's open car, tossing in a grenade that injured him only slightly, but tore through the car's upholstery. Heydrich rallied, but died a week later of either a botulism or anthrax infection acquired from the horse hair–stuffed seats of his car.

By 1980, anthrax had become a favored weapon of modern war—both formally declared conflicts and acts of terrorism. South Africa, for example, unleashed it against Zimbabwe in the Rhodesian civil war.

Investigational Bondage
In response to a Department of Defense application in 1987, the FDA quietly granted the DOD a waiver of informed consent for testing anthrax vaccine.

President Bill Clinton signed Presidential Executive Order 13139 that allows the DOD to experiment on service personnel without their consent or knowledge, *if deemed in the interest of national security.*

This exception allowed the military to test a botulinum toxoid vaccine as well as pyridostigmine bromide tablets as a prophylactic against bioweapons without informed consent. It forced ground troops to take the experimental injections and tablets without being told the intention, track record, or risks of the studies.

Thus, just four decades after the Army oversaw the Nuremberg trial of Nazi physicians on charges that included conducting experiments upon the powerless without their consent, the Department of Defense opted to experiment on its own soldiers without their consent.

An effective, uncontaminated anthrax vaccine with a reasonable ratio of known risks to potential benefits would have been a godsend to soldiers deployed to the Korean Peninsula, Iraq, and other areas where inhalation to deadly anthrax was a possibility. But testing even ideal drug candidates against their will violated not only soldiers' autonomy but also distributive justice, because the risks and the benefits of the research were unevenly distributed: Everyone would benefit from development of a safe, effective vaccine, but only soldiers faced the risks of injury and disease. The government took advantage of their vulnerability as soldiers bound to obey orders and constrained by the Feres doctrine, without legal remedies.

The anthrax testing was also begun four decades after the Army's first disastrous foray into vaccination experiments, the Edgewood Arsenal human experiments, conducted between 1948 and 1975, when the Army Chemical Corps secretly tested 250 pharmaceuticals and vaccines on 7,000 troops. The Army classified the experiments, which prevented injured veterans from seeking medical attention and disability benefits for their exposure to VX, sarin, and mustard gas, as well as to LSD and vaccines. The subsequent lawsuit concluded that the Army had a duty to notify affected veterans of the exposures affecting their health.

But by 1997, Secretary of Defense William Cohen ordered the immunization of all 2.4 million soldiers with the experimental eighteen-month, six-shot inoculation vaccine via its Anthrax Vaccination Immunization Program (AVIP).

Subsequent events seemed to justify the urgency. In June 1993, Aum Shinrikyo, a Japanese doomsday cult, sowed panic by releasing anthrax spores from a Tokyo building. An unclassified DOD report from 1999 alleged that at least ten nations were then developing an offensive capacity to use anthrax in biological warfare: China, Iran, Iraq, Israel, Libya, North Korea, South Korea, Syria, Taiwan, and Russia.

Anthrax also made an occasional domestic-terrorism appearance that decade, as in 1998 when Larry Wayne Harris, linked to the white supremacist group Aryan Nations, was arrested in Nevada while carrying *B. anthracis* spores.

Just a month after the coordinated September 11, 2001, terrorist attacks, a domestic terror campaign deployed anthrax widely and frequently throughout the eastern U.S., largely through the mail. In October, twenty-six Senate staffers and five police officers were exposed to anthrax that was mailed to Senate Majority Leader Tom Daschle. Three Senate office buildings were immediately sealed and decontaminated. But the Brentwood Mail Processing and Distribution Center facility in Washington, D.C., which processed letters contaminated with anthrax, did not close. More than 90 percent of the 2,646 workers there were Black. Four workers at Brentwood fell ill from the anthrax, and two died. Post-9/11 anti-Muslim xenophobia was exacerbated by messages accompanying some of the "anthrax letters" such as "Allah is great" and "Death to America."

Around this time, anthrax spores were detected in the Manhattan office of New York governor George Pataki. He and his staff began taking the antibiotic Cipro, but while New York

City postal workers complained that they feared contamination of the mail and their workplaces, the antibiotic was not made available to them. Anthrax mailed to NBC and a Florida company was tested by the Centers for Disease Control and Prevention, which revealed that the strains were nearly identical: One of the Florida workers died.

Mortality during the anthrax-letter attacks was 45 percent, even with antibiotics and aggressive supportive care.

While anthrax attacks roiled the nation, the anthrax vaccine production was in crisis, too. Serious quality-control issues, including contamination, continuously plagued the Lansing, Michigan, manufacturing facilities of Bioport, the nation's only maker of the anthrax vaccine. From the beginning, Bioport was unable to supply the quality or number of doses that it had promised the DOD. Investigative reports in the *Washington Post* and *Salon* revealed that "because of questions about the facility's quality control," the Pentagon was forced to "dramatically reduce its program to vaccinate all 2.4 million U.S. soldiers and reservists against anthrax."

Soon after the AVIP was initiated, soldiers began complaining of side effects, some so debilitating that troops were unable to function. By October 2001, about 570,000 military personnel had received at least one shot and more than 400 "refusers" had been disciplined for insubordination.

Concerns about serious side effects were voiced by some officers as well as foot soldiers. Throughout his richly varied career, for example, Lt. Col. Russell E. Dingle, a commercial pilot with American Airlines and a flight commander with the Connecticut Air National Guard and then with the Air Force

34   Reserve, advocated for affected soldiers as he wrote and testified
     before judges, members of Congress, the news media—anyone
     in power who would listen—to end the experimentation.

     The Connecticut Air National Guard had initially appointed
     Lt. Col. Dingle to investigate the vaccine. Dingle determined
     that the vaccine was unsafe and ineffective against the airborne
     anthrax spores threatening soldiers—a finding that he said cost
     him his job in the National Guard.

     But the Air Force Reserve subsequently welcomed him and
     he served as a resource for pilots and crew members with con-
     cerns about the vaccine. Until his 2005 death at only forty-five,
     Dingle had spent thousands of hours lobbying, testifying, and
     serving as an anthrax vaccine expert for the U.S. Government
     Accountability Office and the Connecticut attorney general's
     office.

     Investigators found thirty major violations in the manu-
     facturing process by **BioPort**, the vaccine manufacturer, and it
     was shut down by the FDA until January 2002, when it resumed
     operations.

     Yet the punishment of soldiers who resisted taking the
     shots continued.

     Friendly Fire
     One of these was Jemekia Barber. She had refused to undergo
     the vaccinations, but the Army did not need Barber's permis-
     sion. So she consulted a lawyer and tried to resolve the issue
     by requesting a transfer to a unit where she would not need to
     submit to the injections.

     She says her commanding officer blocked it, intending to
     "make an example" of her, and that he encouraged her erstwhile

comrades to harangue her into compliance, shouting in her face, questioning her patriotism, and demanding that she accept the injections. "Not all my comrades confronted me. Some told me in private that they supported me, that they were on my side."

But others were not. "I was bothered by the blatant disrespect of the men around me, who were pushing me as they shouted at me to 'Take the shot!' I'm a small person, and it was deeply troubling." She relates being physically assaulted by a superior officer, followed by confinement to a barracks, a large but empty dormitory building where she had to sign in periodically and was alone except for visits by her commanding officer and an assortment of hostile fellow soldiers—until the day she jumped out of a second-story window and fled:

> I did so because I learned that I was being detained in a building where a gang rape had taken place on the same floor just two weeks earlier. I called my husband saying "Come get me. Now," and when his car pulled up, I just prayed and jumped.

Demoralized and suffering from post-traumatic stress syndrome, she spent time in the brig and in a mental-care facility until, in the end, she accepted the proffered "Chapter 10" hardship discharge that would avoid a court-martial, saying she did so because "they called me the day of my grandfather's funeral presenting this as my only option to leave with dignity. I was assured that I would be given nothing less than an honorable discharge."

But on May 11, 2000, upon recommendation of the battalion commander, she received a less-than-honorable "administrative discharge."

36   Legal briefs note that, "The commander believed that characterization was warranted" because "Barber was manipulative and premeditated in her conduct. She seeks to benefit herself through her misbehavior."

She unsuccessfully appealed the discharge in 2003, by which time her husband had also been released with an administrative discharge, so that the family tradition of military service seems to have suffered a brutal derailment. So did her marriage, the end of which she attributes largely to the stress of fighting the immunizations. "I sometimes wonder what would have happened if we'd never had to fight the shots. But I won't dwell on it."

Physician, Save Thyself
Captain Jon Buck, MD, an emergency physician at Keesler Air Force Base in Biloxi, Mississippi, also refused the vaccine. He objected to the bypassing of informed consent in principle, as he told *Time* in 2001: "There are three foundations in medicine—science, trust, and patient rights—and the mandatory nature of this program violates all three of them."

But he was also deeply concerned about the symptoms of autoimmune disorder, including fatigue and joint pain, that he observed and treated in the wake of anthrax vaccinations, and he didn't want this fate for himself.

"I asked them not to put me in this position because I didn't want something like this to affect my ability to practice medicine for the rest of my life."

Unlike Barber, who was bullied, assaulted, and feared even worse from some of her male peers, Buck said, "My colleagues are in complete support of me, but everybody has to make their own decision."

Even his superior officer, Col. Richard Griffith, said, "I believe he is very sincere, that he believes what he is doing is right. . . . I do not believe he is trying to subvert the mission." Yet in 2001 Buck was court-martialed on a charge of "willfully disobeying a lawful command" where he faced five years in jail, dismissal from the military, and loss of all pay and benefits.

In May 2001, Lt. Col. Dingle, the Air Force Reserve flight commander mentioned above, wrote to members of Congress asking them to intervene in Buck's court-martial:

> When the U.S. military no longer allows for professional dissent within its ranks; when the U.S. military mandates that any and all orders be obeyed regardless of their moral or legal basis; when the U.S. military allows its members to defend themselves with "I was just following orders"; then the U.S. military will cease to attract men and women of principle and honor. . . . It will end up resembling the military organizations that we have fought for the last sixty years.

Like Barber, Buck had requested a conditional resignation that would preclude a dishonorable discharge, and like Barber, he was refused. He was sentenced to sixty days of base restriction, reprimanded, and fined $21,000.

Major Sonnie Bates, a highly decorated thirteen-year veteran Air Force pilot, was the highest-ranking regular-service officer to protest the anthrax vaccine. He drew national attention but ultimately was fined $3,200, was given a general discharge, and lost his military pension.

38   **"Defending the Rights of Others"**

Air Force Col. Leernest Ruffin, who is still on active duty, accepted the vaccine injection series in 2010, just as he had accepted "going to Afghanistan and having to get the malaria medication, which was, you know, some pills that caused bad dreams, hallucinations, all kinds of problems."

In 2010, after reading my book *Medical Apartheid,* Ruffin sent me an email that read in part, "As an Active Duty service member I have often felt like a 'lab rat' especially when the Anthrax shot became mandatory. . . . It seems that our inability to see ourselves in one another can sometimes cause research to go down the wrong road."

When we spoke in 2019, I told him of witnessing constraints on soldiers' behavior as a child. The Army established curfews, declared certain restaurants, bars, and organizations "off limits"; mandated payments to dependent family members; and forced soldiers and pilots to accept medications as part of "fitness for duty" requirements. As a result, I said, "I feel like a cultural climate is created where soldiers are perhaps more likely to accept limitations on their freedom."

Ruffin replied, "Well, I think that's a part of what you do when you raise your right hand. You realize that you are supporting and defending the rights of others and you can't necessarily enjoy those rights yourself."

In 2003, the same year that Barber lost her appeal, a case regarding the legality of the anthrax vaccinations came before Judge Emmet G. Sullivan of the United States District Court in Washington, D.C. If Sullivan's name sounds familiar, that may be because he is the judge who in August 2018 learned that the Trump administration had deported an immigrant mother and daughter who are plaintiffs in a lawsuit over asylum restrictions that he was hearing. In a widely publicized act, Sullivan immediately ordered the government to "turn the plane around and bring those people back to the United States."

Judge Sullivan ruled to end the forced experimental vaccinations. "The women and men of our armed forces put their lives on the line every day to preserve and safeguard the freedoms that all Americans cherish and enjoy. Absent an informed consent or presidential waiver, the United States cannot demand that members of the armed forces also serve as guinea pigs for experimental drugs."

But soldiers' jubilation was short-lived. The FDA responded by granting approval to the experimental anthrax vaccine, instantly elevating it from a questionable investigational drug to an approved therapeutic. This allowed the DOD to sidestep the intent of the decision and to continue forcing the medications on soldiers as part of fitness-for-battle measures.

The FDA approval returned U.S. soldiers to a state of investigative servitude—"investigative" because the data collection and evaluation of the anthrax vaccine risks, including deaths, continued. In rapidly approving the vaccine, the FDA also violated its own regulations by failing to hold the required public hearings.

In the aftermath, the vaccine was demonstrated unsafe. Following complaints at Dover Air Force Base (DAFB), for example, Colonel Felix Grieder, who had suspended the base's vaccination program because of its health hazards, pointed out that the DAFB vaccines were a variant that contained squalene to increase the effectiveness of the vaccines. Squalene is also known to cause the symptoms experienced by Dover soldiers,

40   and a survey of vaccinated unit members showed that 32 per-
      cent suffered severe joint pain, memory loss, and arthritis, a
      much higher-than-average incidence than those reported at
      other military installations.

          The vaccine program's critics also note that squalene's
      side effects mirror the symptoms of Gulf War Syndrome,
      which plagued U.S. soldiers but seemed to spare foreign troops
      fighting in the same theaters of war.

          National evidence surfaced of the vaccine's harms, including
      a 2007 leaked Department of the Army memo entitled, "Tasking
      Order 18-04-01 (Soldier Anthrax Vaccination 2001–2007)." It
      belatedly admitted that vaccinations had harmed some troops
      badly enough to warrant full disability pensions. It read in part,

          The purpose of this tasking informs Soldiers who received
          bad Anthrax batches from Ft. Campbell and Ft. Drum from
          2001–2007 for OEF/OIF IOT notify possible 100 percent VA
          disabilities due to bad anthrax batches.

          At the time, the DOD had dismissed the leaked document
      as a "fake" and a "scam." But in 2018, more than a decade later,
      an independent legal analysis determined the memo "cannot be
      summarily dismissed as fraudulent."

White-Coat Terrorist

In 2010, an FBI investigation that had spanned eight years and
six continents determined that Army microbiologist Bruce E.
Ivins, who worked in a high-security lab at Fort Detrick's pre-
mier biodefense research center, had prepared and mailed the
anthrax spores that killed five people, sickened seventeen others,

generated mass anxiety, and cost the government and private
industry billions to defend the country against anthrax attacks.

But just as shocking is Ivins's motivation for "the worst act of bioterrorism in U.S. history." As the *Washington Post* reported,

> A ninety-six-page summary of the [FBI] investigation concludes that Ivins hatched the anthrax-by-mail scheme in hopes of creating a scare that would rescue what he considered his greatest achievement, an [Army] anthrax vaccine program that he had helped create but that by 2001 was in danger of failing.

The *New York Times* reported:

> [United States attorney Jeffrey] Taylor suggested that Dr. Ivins might have mailed the letters out of concern for the future of an anthrax vaccination program for the military, which was threatened after soldiers had claimed they were sickened by the injections.... Dr. Ivins, who had dedicated his career to the anthrax vaccine, might have plotted the attacks to create "a scenario where people all of a sudden realize the need to have this vaccine."

Thus, in a twist macabre enough for a science-fiction film, the FBI found that the high-ranking Army microbiologist had unleashed anthrax in a mad attempt to save the DOD's program of compulsive immunization based on his own vaccine, which was beginning to be seriously threatened by complaints of illness and contamination.

Ivins committed suicide just before his scheduled 2008 trial, so there exists no legal decision to definitively establish his guilt. Some, including his family, friends, and a 2011 Pro Publica investigation, question the FBI's conclusion.

By a conservative estimate, 2,500 soldiers refused the experimental vaccines and many of these were court-martialed, jailed, or like Barber, were forced out with less-than-honorable discharges. Others fled voluntarily. The General Accounting Office surveyed 829 Air Force pilots and air crews and found that concerns about the safety of the mandatory shots played a role in the decision of 25 percent of them to transfer from or leave the military.

For her part, Barber continued to fight her less-than-honorable discharge on the basis that it was morally wrong to force her to take experimental vaccinations, especially when they were neither safe nor proven effective. Finally, the ruling against her was reversed and she was granted an honorable discharge.

Today she is remarried with a new family, home, and career, so that her determination to escape the oppressive past seems to have borne fruit. Yet in 2019, when I congratulated her on her legal victory, she corrected me, quick as thought.

"I didn't win," she said firmly. Then, in a faltering voice. "I didn't win." She pauses. "I loved the Army." For the first time in all the years I've spoken with her, a quaver invades her voice. "I enjoyed the atmosphere of education and responsibility and the people it attracted, my comrades."

"I still miss it."

The Legacy of Nuremberg

It is the most fundamental tenet of medical ethics and human decency that the subjects volunteer for the experiment after being informed of its nature and hazards. This is the clear dividing line between criminal and what may be noncriminal.
—Andrew Ivy, MD

Informed consent has long been ingrained into U.S. culture as an inalienable right in medical research. To understand why, reflect that many date the inception of modern bioethics from a dramatic confrontation that began on December 9, 1946, at the Palace of Justice in Nuremberg, Germany. Under the aegis of the U.S. Army, American prosecutors confronted the doctors of National Socialism—architects of assault, murder, and genocide masked as human experimentation, all of it forcible.

America vs. Karl Brandt, et al, conducted under military auspices, ended with more than the conviction and punishment of the Nazi doctors. In 1947, it also produced the Nuremberg Code, a set of ethical guidelines for human experimentation. The

44   Allies denounced Nazi experiments conducted on Jews, Poles, Afro-Germans, homosexuals, concentration-camp inmates, and other marginalized groups. These "studies" typically unleashed medical violence including deaths and sought to justify this by invoking emergent conditions, including wartime military expedience. That same year, the U.S. Atomic Energy Commission issued a memo that advocated for stringent informed consent for domestic government-sponsored research.

This military rationale drove Dachau scientists to inflict extensive burns and to immerse subjects in ice-water baths, mimicking the condition of downed German pilots. Physician-researchers explained that they had to quickly find the best way to restore their pilots' body temperature and keep them alive. Researchers also riddled Dachau inmates with gunshots and subjected others to limb amputations without anesthesia, again in order to emulate the plight of wounded soldiers in the field. Once again researchers invoked the need to urgently address the soldiers' welfare and the emergent conditions.

Free Will on Trial
The "Doctors' Trial" was the first and most infamous of the mid-century war-crimes trials. But it also bred a key misconception: that Nazi doctors violated an existing universal code of conduct that mandated voluntary consent, the subject's basic right to freely say *yes* or *no* to involvement in medical research. It's true that the German doctors did not adhere to such a universal code of conduct. But it is also true that this universal code of conduct was only invented during their trial; they were then accused of violating it. During the trial, Andrew Ivy, the American Medical Association representative, alluded to U.S. principles on medical

ethics in human experimentation to which Germans had failed to adhere, but when questioned, he had to admit that the principles in question had been devised only on December 28, 1946, in anticipation of his testimony at the Doctors' Trial.

Prior to this, the legal requirement to offer informed consent to all subjects did exist—but only in Germany. The idea of consent to research had informed American research ethics and law since the 1830s, but U.S. federal consent principles were very inconsistently applied and rarely formally written until the Nuremberg Code was devised.

In the early twentieth century, German physicians occupied the apex of the medical profession. They had designed stringent ethical codes that required informed consent. But by mid-century, the abuses they perpetrated illustrated that no matter how clear and potent on paper, rules and laws don't protect subjects if they are ignored, and their violations are rationalized and unpunished.

The U.S. should have taken heed of this hypocrisy, because we, too, have fallen victim to it. Despite today's rich matrix of federal laws and professional codes, we have frequently abandoned informed consent and today remain guilty of burgeoning medical experimentation without consent of any type.

One reason why we have failed to consistently provide the informed consent promised by the Code and its successors is that shortly after its adoption, the Nuremberg Code's idealism was eclipsed for U.S. researchers by the less constricting World Medical Association's Code of Ethics, the Declaration of Helsinki. "The World Medical Association interpreted the Nuremberg Code so it was responsive to the needs of the practice," writes Yale bioethicist Robert J. Levine. According to his late

46   Yale colleague Jay Katz, American scientists saw the Nuremberg Code as a good code for barbarians but an unnecessary code for ordinary physicians.

Moreover, twentieth-century U.S. and German scientists also embraced eugenics. The term, coined by Francis Galton, a cousin of Charles Darwin, applied to beliefs first ascendant between 1900 and 1910, when geneticists discovered human traits that adhered to a Mendelian pattern of inheritance. In this pattern, the breeding of two carrier parents resulted in a mathematically predictable mixture of well, ill, and carrier offspring. The birth of an affected child from unaffected parents signaled that the parents were carriers.

Galton used this knowledge to propose the desirability of using selective procreation to refine the human race while conquering social dysfunction. By the 1930s, this goal was widely and enthusiastically embraced on both scientific and popular levels, first in the United States, then abroad, notably in Germany. Eugenics was applied to not only entire groups but also done to individual human beings.

The "unfit" races were deemed "swarthy," "black," "ugly." Flattened noses, wiry black hair, and prognathous profiles characterized the "lower" ethnicities and such depictions were used to popularize eugenics. Eugenics fit well within the framework of racial discrimination and ideas of inferiority, as it provided biological, pseudoscientific justification for such prejudices that were common in the U.S. and Germany. Eugenic yardsticks were devised and applied to not only populations but also to individuals.

Eugenicists proposed that society use medical information about disease and trait inheritance to end social ills by encouraging the birth of children with good, healthy, and beautiful traits. This was positive eugenics, but the movement also had a negative face: eugenicists promulgated the weeding out of undesirable societal elements by discouraging or preventing their reproduction.

Eugenics dovetailed nicely with racial and ethnic biases, offering a biological scaffold for the strong beliefs in hereditary racial inferiority that were shared by the United States and Germany. Their scientists worked closely on eugenic initiatives and research, and eugenicists invoked the term *racial hygiene* as frequently as they did *eugenics*. Even a cursory glance at the charts, photographs, and diagrams used to popularize eugenic ideals reveals that the unfit were "swarthy," "black," and ugly by Anglo-Saxon standards, with flattened noses, wiry black hair, and prognathous profiles.

Moreover, historian Robert Proctor reminds us that doctors invented racial hygiene: It was not imposed on them. Eugenics moved from "positive" to "negative" goals like actively seeking to remove pollutant genetic "inferiors"—including Jews and Blacks—from the gene pool. By 1929, before Hitler took the reins, 3,000 doctors belonged to the Nazi party. In 1934, Rudolf Hess summarized: "National Socialism is nothing but applied biology." By 1942, the number of Nazi doctors had swelled to 38,000, as Jews were methodically excluded from medical practice, and men and women with African heritage were forcibly sterilized. Those purged from the German gene pool included the children of German women and French African soldiers in the Rheinland as well as some offspring of colonial German soldiers and Herero women living in what is now Namibia.

But at the Doctors' Trial, Karl Brandt, MD, did not defend German researchers by invoking fading eugenic precepts.

48   Instead, he charged Americans with committing the very same crimes of dangerous and coerced research, also in the name of military expedience, that they decried in Nazi physicians.

A member of the German defense team read verbatim into the trial transcript a 1945 *Life* magazine article describing the U.S. Army wartime experiments on eight hundred prisoners at the Stateville Penitentiary near Joliet, Illinois. The University of Chicago Department of Medicine had conducted the experiment in conjunction with the United States Army and the State Department.

Quinine, the standard of care, was largely unavailable and researchers cited an urgent need for new malaria treatments. U.S. soldiers were deployed to areas of the Pacific with extremely high rates of malaria infection, and when the inevitable illness set in, they were administered untested drugs under controlled conditions to evaluate the agents' safety and effectiveness. They were neither told they were part of an experiment nor given the opportunity to refuse the drugs.

Ivy's defense claimed that such American subjects had never been abused or used involuntarily, but he must have known better: Dr. Ivy himself had been involved in the malaria experiments performed with the Illinois State Penitentiary inmates. And just a year after Nuremberg, the *Journal of the American Medical Association* praised the experiments.

Yet during the trial, Ivy testified:

It is the most fundamental tenet of medical ethics and human decency that the subjects volunteer for the experiment after being informed of its nature and hazards. This is the clear dividing line between criminal and what may be noncriminal.

If the experimental subjects cannot be said to have volunteered, then the inquiry need proceed no further.

Judgment in the Doctors' Trial was handed down on August 19, 1947, and included imprisonment and death for the Nazi physicians.

The trial served not only to expose and punish the Third Reich's atrocities, murders, and crimes against humanity in the name of medical research, but also afforded an opportunity to craft a global standard for research ethics and human rights so that no one could ever be forced into research servitude again.

Unfortunately, the U.S. has come to ignore Nuremberg's uncompromising insistence on informed consent as "emergency conditions" and military expedience have been invoked to weaken present-day Americans' right to say *yes* or *no* to becoming medical research subjects.

The medical crimes that were denounced and punished at Nuremberg have American analogues. Although not perfect parallels, they share a violent, nonconsensual, and largely racial disparate nature, as well as the frequent invocation of military expedience.

NAZI RESEARCH	US RESEARCH
FREEZING EXPERIMENTS	INDUCED HYPOTHERMIA
Until 1942, German Air Force doctors at Dachau seeking the best way to warm flyers who landed in frigid waters forced naked camp inmates to stand in freezing weather for up to fourteen hours and submerged others in ice-water tanks for three-hour periods.	In recent years, physicians in various medical institutions intentionally induced *profound hypothermia* by infusing cold saltwater solution into a subject's blood vessels until his core temperature plummets dangerously. Researchers' speculation that oft-fatal hypothermia may discourage brain damage has yet to be demonstrated.

50

NAZI RESEARCH	US RESEARCH
MALARIA	MALARIA
Malariotherapy is an experimental technique that has long sought to treat other infections such as syphilis and HIV by inducing malaria in hopes that the resultant high fevers will kill pathogens. About 1,200 healthy Dachau inmates were subjected to repeated bites by or injected matter from malaria-infected mosquitoes. The rationale was to test remedies including quinine, neosalvarsan, pyramidon, and antipyrine. Approximately four hundred of the subjects died of malaria or its complications.	Malariotherapy was used in the 1930s by Dr. Mark Boyd and in the 1980s by Dr. Henry Heimlich, the popularizer of the "Heimlich maneuver," who conducted malariotherapy in the United States, Ethiopia, Malawi, and China. The research study "Malaria Challenge With NF54 Strain," done between 2009 and 2011, was designed to subject thirty-eight volunteers to repeated bites from mosquitoes until they became infected. As with the German experiment, the rationale was to test candidate vaccines. The study site was heavily Black Baltimore, using *p. falciparum,* the most deadly North American strain of malaria. The FDA and CDC denounce malariotherapy as dangerous.
SEA-WATER (SALINE) EXPERIMENTS	HYPERTONIC SALINE EXPERIMENTS
In July 1944, German military experimented with nonconsenting Roma ("gypsies") at Dachau. They claimed that they sought how best to render sea water potable in order to help soldiers and sailors trapped in areas without drinking water. But the experimental subjects were given 1) untreated saltwater, 2) saltwater whose salt content was retained, although the brackish taste had been eliminated, 3) no water at all, and 4) desalinated water, given only to one group. The expectation was that most would die.	In ongoing nonconsensual ROC (Resuscitation Outcomes Consortium) experiments that target urban areas, highly concentrated saltwater was infused into blood vessels from 2006 until 2008, when the study was suspended in the wake of Data and Safety Monitoring Board (DSMB) concerns.
JEWISH SKELETON COLLECTIONS	AFRICAN-AMERICAN SKELETAL CACHES
One hundred and fifteen subjects, seventy-nine of them Jewish, were murdered in order to round out a Nazi collection of racial skulls, which	In 1995, 9,800 bones, 75 percent of them from African Americans, were discovered sealed beneath the floors of the Medical College of Georgia's former

NAZI RESEARCH	US RESEARCH
JEWISH SKELETON COLLECTIONS (CONT.) Dr. Wolfram Sievers, director of the Institute for Military Scientific skulls. In 1943–44, the corpses were sent to Strasbourg for processing, but in 1944, fearing the collection's discovery by advancing Allied forces, they were dissolved, presumably in acid. Some skeleton fragments remain.	AFRICAN-AMERICAN SKELETAL CACHES (CONT.) anatomy laboratory. Similar caches of such discarded "training material" have been unearthed, and occasionally displayed, at US university medical centers.
HIGH-ALTITUDE EXPERIMENTS In 1942, Sigmund Rascher, a physician and captain in the German Air Force at Dachau, locked subjects into a pressure chamber in order to simulate extremely high altitudes, as high as forty-seven thousand feet, and changing them very rapidly, mimicking the conditions that would befall a pilot in freefall without oxygen or a parachute. The researchers wrote dispassionate reports, including "necropsies" of subjects while their hearts were still beating.	DEEP-DIVING EXPERIMENTS In 1981, Duke University's Atlantis III experiment sent three experienced divers into a pressure chamber that simulated a thirty-six-day dive to 2,250 feet, then a new world record. The informed consent process warned them of the risks of joint pain, disability, and other injuries, including death. But in a lawsuit filed by one of the divers, neither the researcher nor the informed-consent form warned of the danger of the permanent organic brain damage that the subject suffered. The courts excused Duke, calling profound brain damage an unforeseeable risk.
BURNS FROM INCENDIARY BOMBS In November 1943, researchers burned five Buchenwald inmates with phosphorus taken from bombs.	RADIATION BURNS In 1947, the nation's first civilian burn unit at the Medical College of Virginia, funded by the Army, selectively burned African-American subjects to discern whether radiation burns would be deeper or more severe than those induced on skins of whites. They focused beams of light to simulate the "flash burn" an individual could receive from a nuclear blast. Researchers deduced that Blacks suffered more intense burns than whites after the same exposure and concluded that radiation from a nuclear event would injure Blacks much more severely than whites.

NAZI RESEARCH	US RESEARCH
INFECTIONS From 1942 to 1943, one hundred nonconsenting concentration-camp subjects were injected with an experimental typhus vaccine, then some were intentionally exposed to the virus. Inmates were also exposed to yellow fever, smallpox, paratyphoid, cholera, and diphtheria. Other subjects were kept infected with typhus in order to provide a pool of contagious material.	**INFECTIOUS AND RADIOACTIVE ELEMENTS** Historian Susan Lederer notes that US physicians have infected subjects with infectious diseases on at least forty occasions since 1892. An experimental group of 460 Black and 770 white patients at the Medical College of Virginia was injected with a variety of radioactive substances, including phosphorus-32, without their consent. *The Plutonium Files* describes another program in which about eighteen unwitting patients were injected with plutonium and monitored for years.
BONE, MUSCLE, AND NERVE REGENERATION AND TRANSPLANTATION Doctors Fritz Fischer and Herta Oberheuser of Ravensbrück simulated battle injuries by making incisions in women's legs, into which they inserted glass shards or wood chips. Later they shot the inmates or simulated bullet wounds by tying off small blood vessels, provoked gangrene by inserting gangrene cultures, and tested various surgical and medical remedies, including sulfanilamide. Researchers also transplanted bones and tissues between inmates.	**BLOOD AND TISSUE TRANSPLANTATION** Between 1951 and 1974, Dr. Albert Kligman conducted research at Philadelphia's Holmesburg Prison in which foreign tissues were implanted into the backs of prisoners to test transplantation techniques. Most subjects were Black. The first US cases of solid-organ transplants featured organ appropriation from nonconsenting Black patients into white subjects. Blood, the body's largest organ, was used to make some contemporary HBOC blood substitutes, including PolyHeme, that were tested without informed consent.

False Blood

Never ask when you can take.
Ferengi Rule of Acquisition No. 52,
Star Trek Memory Alpha

Martha Milete welcomed Carlos into her Detroit home on a blustery January evening. "We'd finished dinner and gone into the bedroom," Martha told me. "Then, as we disrobed, we heard a thump. A loud one."

It was probably nothing, Martha thought, maybe a dog in the street outside. She rose to open the bedroom door, and found herself staring at two men brandishing large handguns. One of the masked intruders held a gun against her temple as the duo shoved her and Carlos back into the dining room and thrust them, naked, onto their knees, snarling at them to keep their hands behind their heads. As one thug batted drawers open and pawed through sideboards and chests, the other barked, "Give me all the money, all you've got."

"But I had no money, and I told them, 'There's nothing in the house.'" Looking around her tastefully decorated home, they seemed not to believe her.

"Yes, you do," the first invader said slowly and distinctly, his gun trained on her.

"I looked into his eyes: They were dead. And suddenly I knew. I knew. I begged him, 'Don't! Please don't! Don't hurt me. Don't shoot me' I was still begging him when I was blown backward by the force of the gun's blast. I couldn't breathe and felt a searing pain in my eye. They ran through the front door.

"Carlos kneeled over me, and applied pressure to my chest, trying to stanch the bleeding. He pressed his hand over my chest, shouting for help, for what seemed like a long time, but no one came. I could tell he was scared and suddenly, he stood up and ran away, too. I was alone.

"I couldn't see much, but I was able to call my son, Jason, on my cell phone and say 'I've been shot' before everything went black.

"Jason called 9-1-1. He saved my life."

The ambulance screamed to her home, and Martha remembers that in the ambulance, "I woke up. I was conscious while an EMT gave me blood, but then I passed out and I don't remember anything after that until I was in the hospital."

Minutes after her son's frantic 9-1-1 call, Martha lay in Detroit's Sinai Grace hospital, where she underwent a six-hour bout of surgery, the first of many, for the gunshot wound to her chest. She had become another victim of U.S. urban gun violence, one of one hundred thousand Americans shot in 2006.

For days, Martha hovered between a vestigial conscious-ness and oblivion. "I would come to in the hospital and hear a little conversation, and then I'd black out again. They had me strapped down for two or three days and for days, two people—a guy and a girl—kept drawing blood from me: At first I thought it was part of the hospital routine.

"When I became a little more alert, I realized that the people who were drawing blood were not part of the team caring for me. For one thing, they wore insignia that read 'Wayne State University' and all they wanted was my blood. They were taking blood twice a day and wanted more; they were just standing in the doorway waiting for more blood, both of them. I remember getting real upset one day: I was starting to feel a little better, and realizing what was going on, I said, 'You're not taking one more ounce of blood from me. Stop and leave me alone.'

"Then my daughter Cathy told me why, that it was part of the medical experiment that I was in. She explained that when I was bleeding heavily, lying between life and death, they had given me an experimental liquid instead of blood, the artificial blood. It was called PolyHeme."

Did no one from the hospital or research team tell her that she had been enrolled in the experiment? "No, my daughter told me. The medical staff never told me. They were still studying me as part of an experiment. There was a coordinator who kept telling nurses to 'take more blood, take more blood.' She was in cahoots with the research people.

"I could not believe it! I told them that I wanted no part of it. It was wrong. Although I survived, it was wrong. How can they make you a guinea pig without asking your permission?"

How indeed? Because, as Chapter Seven will explain, in the fall of 1996, everyday U.S. residents had joined prisoners and soldiers in becoming research subjects without their consent. Martha's experience was sanctioned by the 1996 addendum to the Code of Federal Regulations: specifically, statute 21 CFR 50.24.

Without her knowledge, she was enrolled in an experimental study of the blood substitute PolyHeme, which was infused in a study involving 720 unwitting U.S. and Canadian research subjects between 2003–2006 by EMTs on ambulances.

Why a blood substitute? Because whether rent by gunshots, steering wheels, or blown aneurysms, the torn bodies of trauma victims crave blood. When an ambulance arrives at a trauma scene, replacing the blood ebbing from the victim's body becomes a priority because lost blood volume can send a person into shock. The body depends upon hemoglobin, the scarlet protein that enables red blood cells to ferry oxygen throughout the body. Too much lost blood, unreplaced for too long, starves tissues and organs, including the brain, of oxygen, resulting in unconsciousness, organ damage, and finally death. Thus, a blood transfusion replenishes fading tissues with fluid and oxygen and it is the best, safest proven treatment for hemorrhaging trauma victims.

But ambulances cannot slake the thirst of injured bodies with blood, because blood can take an hour to type and match, and it requires refrigeration and space to store the necessary variety of types. Type O negative, the so-called "universal donor," is no panacea: It is rare and less than universal because its antibodies may evoke dangerous reactions during a transfusion. Ambulances find blood too expensive—in time, space, and money—to store.

Fortunately, a cheap, plentiful, and portable blood substitute has been proven effective and safe: salt water. A solution of 0.9 percent saline, called "normal" because it mimics the saltwater concentration within our bodies, can be quickly and easily infused into trauma victims. Saline solution expands the volume of blood, staving off shock long enough to get the urban or suburban victim to the hospital where blood is available—a trip that typically takes less than twenty minutes.

In residential communities and on city streets, saline is the safe, proven, pre-hospital standard of care. But not for soldiers in the field. For battlefield casualties who are hours from blood and hospital care, saline solution has a critical limitation: It lacks hemoglobin. This leaves the tissues and brains of battlefield victims oxygen-starved for too long and at risk for a cascade of vascular disasters leading to stroke, heart attack, and death.

For decades, the U.S. Department of Defense, acutely aware of the danger to injured soldiers, has been experimenting with different types of blood substitutes, including a freeze-dried "blood" powder that only requires mixing with water and the oxygen-saturated perfluorocarbons that inspired the breathable liquid used by the divers in the film *The Abyss*.

PolyHeme is a different category of blood substitute that is often called *hemoglobin-based oxygen carriers*, or HBOCs. The military's interest and influence extends far beyond contributing subjects and funds to HBOC development: In 2006, Dr. Peter Lurie, MD, of Public Citizen, successfully sued the FDA to stop it from holding illegal closed-door hearings with the Navy in reference to HBOC studies.

Colonel John Holcomb, until 2008 the commander of the Army Institute of Surgical Research on the campus of the

58 Brooke Army Medical Center in San Antonio, has been one of the most aggressive supporters of HBOC research. Holcomb is now a medical consultant for CellPhire, a Maryland biotechnology company whose products include a freeze-dried blood product for trauma care, but in 2007 the *New York Times* reported that he "strongly advocates conducting clinical trials to improve trauma care"—trials of PolyHeme in particular. Holcomb explained that he allowed the center to participate in the trial because PolyHeme seemed safe. Informational materials prepared by the Brooke Center on his watch reassured local communities that, "Up to now, PolyHeme has not caused any clinically bad problems."

But this is untrue. In 1998, PolyHeme had been tested in hospital patients undergoing surgery for aortic aneurysms in the Acute Normovolemic Hemodilution, or ANH, study. Its results were disastrous. Instead of prolonging their lives, ten of eighty-one patients who received the blood substitute suffered a heart attack within seven days, and two of those died. By contrast, none of the seventy-one patients in the trial who received real blood, the hospital standard of care, suffered a heart attack.

"[Holcomb] knew about this data, and he should never have approved the trial for his center and allowed the Army to participate in it," said Keith Berman, editor of *International Blood/ Plasma News*, who has long specialized in research on blood substitutes. Holcomb similarly championed the experimental use of another blood-derived product called Factor VII or NovoSeven, devised to help the blood of hemophiliacs clot—even though it is not FDA-approved for people without clotting disorders.

According to the *New York Times*, Dr. Andrew F. Shorr, a former military physician and now the associate director of

critical care medicine at Washington Hospital Center, believed
that Holcomb "pushed military surgeons to use Factor VII
despite a lack of data on its benefits—and some evidence that it
can increase the risk of blood clots that cause strokes."

Today's obsession with finding a blood substitute con-
tinues a long medical quest. In the seventeenth century, famed
astronomer, mathematician-physicist, and anatomist Christopher Wren infused wine into a dog's bloodstream, and two centuries later, American gynecologist Gaillard Thomas flushed
milk into the veins of pallid postsurgical patients. But no substitutes derived from human blood were tested until 1933, when
William Ruthrauff Amberson of the University of Tennessee
boldly infused hemolyzed (ruptured) red blood into human
patients, which stemmed the flow of urine, provoked brady-
cardia (a dangerously slowed heartbeat), and drove up blood
pressure, culminating in deaths from kidney failure.

By the 1990s, as wars and rumors of wars fed fears that U.S.
battlefield trauma and deaths—which total over 50,000 injuries
from hostile fire in Iraq and Afghanistan alone—would escalate,
the DOD turned its attention to the HBOC blood substitutes.

A 2008 *JAMA* meta-analysis found that HBOCs were ineffective, deadly, or both: Only one, Hemopure, ever gained approval
for human use, and that only in South Africa.

This is because HBOCs share devastating medical limitations: Hemoglobin carries oxygen throughout the body,
but once sprung from the prison of its blood-cell mem-
brane, an unrestrained hemoglobin molecule becomes a rogue
agent tiny enough to indiscriminately penetrate the walls of
veins and arteries. There, free hemoglobin molecules trigger

60   inflammation, causing the muscular cell membranes to seize
      and contract, or they block a blood vessel to the heart, trig-
      gering a heart attack. Studies of one HBOC, HemAssist, had to
      be shut down in 1998 when nearly half of the fifty-two trauma
      patients infused with it died, compared to only 17 percent who
      received standard therapy.

      Each HBOC manufacturer claimed to have generated its
      own unique process to transform free hemoglobin into some-
      thing that can safely carry oxygen; these efforts were not suc-
      cessful, nor have they received approval from the FDA. The term
      "definitively" modified HBOCs is commonly used but entirely
      misleading.

      Milk and wine may seem arcane blood-substitute candi-
      dates, but PolyHeme is made from no less Gothic a substance—
      expired human blood, originally donated for transfusion, but
      long past its shelf life.

      Like the firms before it, Northfield Laboratories, the Evan-
      ston, Illinois, biotechnology company that makes PolyHeme,
      claimed to have discovered the secret ingredient: polymers. By
      rearranging hemoglobin into a chain of quadrupled bundles,
      called tetramers, Northfield claims to have tamed free hemo-
      globins, removing the risk of excess heart attacks and death.
      Northfield CEO Stephen Gould told its stockholders that his
      product would tap into a $1 billion market.

      Northfield's website also celebrated its coziness with the
      military: "Northfield's collaboration with the U.S. Army dates
      back to 1969. We are currently exploring the potential use of
      PolyHeme® in patients in shock in remote battlefield settings,
      where red blood cells are not available."

Northfield claimed that HBOC would benefit civilians, too, by allowing hospitals to avoid time-consuming blood typing, and by replacing real blood in surgeries—a boon to groups like Jehovah's Witnesses, whose religious beliefs proscribe blood transfusions. The latter claim is questionable, however, because PolyHeme is made from human blood.

And like real blood, the HBOC requires refrigeration for optimal storage, although its shelf life is measured in years, not weeks, so it, unlike blood, could be carried on ambulances.

What PolyHeme cannot do is save patients and hospitals money: In fact, it is more expensive and far more profitable than the real blood from which it is made. By 2016, blood products made up 1.9 percent of all American exports, outstripping soybeans.

But before PolyHeme could enter the market, it needed FDA approval. The FDA gives studies just a few years to collect data, and the process of eliciting informed consent is time-consuming, costly, and uncertain. It is easy to understand that for-profit companies such as Northfield would be eager to dispense with informed consent if it stood between them and the FDA approval they require. Mary K. Pendergast, who was with the FDA when the 50.24 exception was adopted, says Poly-Heme researchers favored opt-out studies because, "Practically speaking, otherwise it takes too long."

Companies like Northfield pay the FDA: Since 1992, federal law mandates that corporations pay approximately 40 percent of the cost of evaluating clinical trial data that result in their drugs' approval or rejection. In a clear conflict of interest, that money can occlude medical judgment and hobble FDA independence.

Gould took Northfield public in 1994, then raised $194 million by selling shares to the public. He then turned his attention to convincing the FDA that he had an effective, safe blood substitute. When the disastrous 1998 ANH hospital study of PolyHeme produced excess death and illness, Northfield quietly closed the trial and the company's press releases did not mention the deaths and heart attacks: Gould allayed shareholder anxiety by explaining that Northfield had closed the study because it was progressing too slowly.

However, Northfield could not hide the investigational carnage from the FDA, so Gould claimed that PolyHeme itself was safe, but that the study doctors had bungled the trial by infusing patients with excess fluid.

The doctors could not defend themselves because Northfield withheld data about the entire study from them and did not publish it in peer-reviewed medical journals. Instead, Northfield communicated cherry-picked study data via upbeat press releases and issued gag orders to researchers.

This *omerta* extends to members of the press. *San Diego Reader* investigative reporter Matt Potter described being shunned by nervous PolyHeme researchers who feared that his investigative bent would not produce the uncritically laudatory press that was being generated by other local news media. I myself spent six weeks in an unsuccessful quest to speak with a Northfield official after an initial conversation with communications officer Sophie Twaddell. She demanded, "What is the slant of the article you are writing? What will it say?" After I declined to promise rosy coverage, my phone calls and emails went unreturned for weeks. I was finally given an appointment

for a telephone interview with Gould, which Twaddell canceled
by email on the day it was to take place.

By 2003, the clock was ticking on PolyHeme's patent: The
longer it took Northfield to procure FDA approval, the less time
it would have to enjoy exclusive profits from its sale. But how
could the company hope to entice subjects into a clinical trial
when the tenets of informed consent require that researchers
tell prospective subjects of the heart attacks, deaths, and injuries from the earlier ANH study? How could Northfield persuade
ill or injured people to accept the infusion of a troubled experimental product made from old, expired blood into their veins?

Under normal conditions, two groups of subjects might
have accepted these long odds: people living in rural areas and
soldiers, for whom saline solution, the standard of care, is inadequate to sustain life and health over the long periods before
they can reach a hospital and access to blood. These isolated
conditions alter the risk-benefit ratio.

Yet, except for the Army's Institute of Surgical Research
in San Antonio under PolyHeme-booster Holcomb, PolyHeme
studies used civilians living near hospitals, not rural dwellers or
soldiers.

Twaddell explained that testing under battlefield conditions is impossible. "The Army did it once with hemostatic bandages and they couldn't keep track of them—they got lost," she
said in a magazine interview. "It's very hard to keep data when
people are shooting at you."

This rationale is unconvincing. The history of U.S. medical
research is replete with studies that were conducted successfully

64   under combat and other chaotic conditions, including the successful testing, by Marines, of chitosan bandages and the testing of steroids for head injuries.

There is a far more convincing reason: As Chapter One related, it was the military that fired the first modern legal salvo against informed consent around 1990, in the shadow of an impending Gulf War. A bitter legal fallout from an anthrax vaccine testing study and other cases of forcible experimentation among ground troops ensued. When involuntary experiments with soldiers was banned, many filed lawsuits. Some have been won; others remain active.

So, although defense appropriations for PolyHeme totaled $4.9 million by mid-2006, the DOD's legal reversals—to say nothing of the broken trust between researchers and soldiers— made forcing PolyHeme upon soldiers problematic.

But the 1996 amendment to CFR 21 50.24 permitted Northfield to skirt informed consent with civilians just as the DOD had done with the armed forces. It permitted research without consent on trauma victims with the rationale that something must urgently be done to save their lives.

This law allowed researchers to force PolyHeme upon unconscious accident victims, and thus it was that EMTs who flew to Martha's house in response to her son's anguished call first took the time to open a manila envelope containing a randomly generated computer printout that told them which fluid—saline or PolyHeme—to infuse into the next trauma victim they encountered. The digital coin toss came up PolyHeme.

Martha thinks her ethnicity was a factor. "I know that in Detroit it was used mostly on Black people." The *Detroit Free*

Press reported that fifteen of the sixteen subjects who were driven to Detroit Receiving and Sinai-Grace hospitals in ambulances were Black and Hispanic, including the two subjects who died. "We African Americans have been treated like guinea pigs," said Reverend Charles Williams, president of the National Council for Community Empowerment of Detroit, who organized demonstrations protesting racial disparity in medical research. "We have suffered a history of research abuse and this is yet another instance."

So do demographic data that buttress a racial-bias case against the PolyHeme studies, which enrolled 720 patients in 32 initial research centers across the United States. (At least five centers later dropped out of the trial, citing discomfort with its conduct and protocols.)

In 2006, 10 percent of the more than 3,000 counties in the U.S. had "majority-minority" populations, where ethnic minorities make up more than 50 percent of the populace. But of the municipalities where ambulances carry PolyHeme, 34 percent were majority-minority. Richmond, Virginia, was 57 percent Black; Memphis, Tennessee, was 61 percent Black; Macon, Georgia, was 62 percent Black; and Detroit was then 84 percent Black. The handful of rural sites, like the village of Maywood, Illinois, was 83 percent Black. Of the cities that ultimately completed the trial, thirteen—65 percent—had Black populations considerably higher than the national African-American representation of 13 percent, and some had disproportionately high Hispanic populations, as well.

Even some cities that are not majority-minority employed recruitment schemes that targeted people of color. Using the California Public Records Act, Potter of the *San Diego Reader* found

66   that only ambulances that routinely trolled some Black and Hispanic neighborhoods were selected to distribute PolyHeme.

"Within the city of San Diego, the experiment is targeted at several neighborhoods south of I-8, where many poor and minority residents are unlikely to have heard of the study," Potter wrote.

Federal law normally requires that hospitals and researchers, such as Northfield representatives, collect racial data on their subjects. "But for private companies it is unclear whether they are required to keep such data," observed Heather Butts, former regulatory specialist for Columbia University Medical Center's IRB.

Because Northfield received DOD funds, she suggests, "I would be surprised if they did not collect these ethnic data." If so, I found no evidence that it shared them with the public. Instead, Northfield invoked patient-privacy laws or cited its need to protect "proprietary" information. I did discover data for one testing institution that revealed most subjects were members of ethnic minority groups.

Despite the racially disproportionate recruitment, whites certainly were used as well; in fact it is likely that although ethnic minority members were often used in greater percentages than whites, white subjects remained a numerical majority.

Lawyer Nancy King, a bioethicist at the Wake Forest University who lives in a targeted community and could have been forced into the study, coauthored "An Open Letter to IRBs Considering Northfield Laboratories' PolyHeme Trial," which detailed her concerns. She discovered, for example, that the PolyHeme study violated her state's Patient's Bill of Rights, which guarantees informed consent to anyone participating in medical research.

As a result, the PolyHeme study was suspended in North Carolina as the IRB that had approved it considered the ethical question of impressing citizens into medical research. But the study soon resumed after the bothersome guarantee of informed consent was waived.

PolyHeme provided an example of how a study could be legal yet unethical. But it may not have been legal after all, because the experiment violated several of the conditions that federal law imposes on nonconsensual research.

Nonconsensual studies are bound by a requirement that the subjects' medical condition and time constraints must preclude eliciting informed consent from them or their authorized representatives—and this is usually taken to mean that the subject is unconscious or not lucid enough to give meaningful consent *and* that no family member can be reached without a time lapse that would prove a danger to the subject. However, not every trauma victim is unconscious.

Recall that Martha awoke in the ambulance long enough to watch PolyHeme being infused into her veins. She was conscious, yet the PolyHeme study made no provision for giving conscious subjects the opportunity to give or withhold consent. Or even for determining whether they were indeed unconscious.

"Most reasonable people would want to be informed," observes Peter Lurie, MD, of Public Citizen. "Has anyone actually done the research to establish that this is infeasible? The company will complain that it is too difficult; this doesn't make it impossible."

Another condition is that the experimental modality can be given only when the standard of care, blood, is unavailable.

68   But the PolyHeme protocol violates this tenet, too, by stipu-
lating that PolyHeme must be administered for twelve hours,
more than eleven hours after most of the vast majority of subjects arrive at the hospital, where blood, the hospital standard
of care, is available. This practice violates the condition of a
setting where the standard of care is unsatisfactory or unavailable and in the words of King, "In a hospital, blood is neither."

Why then is PolyHeme infused for a full twelve hours?
Because, King suggests, in order to counter the paucity of military subjects, "The study itself is trying to replicate battlefield
conditions."

As an additional condition, Northfield was directed to devise
a way for people to opt out of the study. The company designed a
bright-blue plastic bracelet inscribed with the words, "I decline
the Northfield PolyHeme study" in big block letters. One can
imagine that this adornment was as unwelcome on formal occa-
sions as on intimate ones, but only by wearing the bracelet
twenty-four hours a day throughout the years of the study's
enrollment period could a trauma victim in the participating
cities expect to escape the study. The catch, of course, is that
you must first have heard of the study and know you are a potential subject.

But most people living in targeted cities never learned of
the PolyHeme study, as I have seen firsthand over more than a
decade, as I've traveled the country to give lectures about the
ethical conduct of medical research. When I speak at a city that
was a PolyHeme research site, I ask if anyone in the audience,
which typically contains hundreds of people, has heard of the
PolyHeme study. Rarely is a hand raised.

Records on file at the FDA demonstrate that those who did appear at "community-notification" meetings received rosy reassurances from investigators via standardized PowerPoint slides, including:

Q: Is PolyHeme safe?

A: In clinical trials to date, PolyHeme® has demonstrated no "clinically relevant" adverse effects. That is, they didn't impact the patient's safety or recovery.

This would surely have been news to the ANH study heart-attack victims—and its dead—who received PolyHeme.

Participating medical center public-relations offices released laudatory releases that ignored the significant risks of HBOCs in general and of PolyHeme in particular. Press materials portrayed PolyHeme as a promising new treatment rather than a troubled experimental product. These were often parroted by local news media.

In the community notification model, the opinion of the group is supposed to be solicited, but the protocol language leaves it unclear whether this feedback could mandate change in the conduct of the trial or whether meeting attendees registering dissent could result in its closure. This proved a moot issue because the PolyHeme community consent meetings presented the study as a fait accompli. Not only was criticism not solicited during conduct of meetings but researchers' comments make it clear that any criticisms made the skeptic a target. Researchers wrote in the margins of the

70   pages that attendees who asked hard questions were "hostile,"
and the "proof" of the few endorsements that they presented
to the FDA were just positive evaluations of the presenters'
performance.

Even the shorthand that researchers adopt to refer to studies
without consent is opaque to laypersons—"EFIC studies," for
"exception from informed consent." Of course it's not just
detailed informed consent that EFIC studies deny subjects like
Martha; they are not afforded any type of consent whatever.

This is just one example of jargon that operates to mini-
mize risks or even to deceive research subjects. Among the most
important are word choices like *patient, treatment,* and *therapy*
that reinforce the illusion that subjects are receiving novel care
rather than being used to test untried approaches.

Community consultation embraced a plethora of troubling assumptions, beginning, as Karla Holloway has noted,
with the very definition of *community.* The urban communities in question were usually ethnically distinctive, poor, and
considered as a monolithic entity for whom blanket notification was sufficient. There was an assumption that a miniscule
sample of the affected population was a reasonable proxy for
a large heterogenous community. Prepared PowerPoint slides
using a template that did not vary from site to site, carefully
choreographed and edited talks, and reassuring appearances
by the people who would be conducting and sponsoring the
trial were accepted as substitutes for eliciting subjects' consent. Besides omitting references to PolyHeme's troubling
past, the presentations deployed jargon and focused on medical urgency that confused attendees about the experimental

nature of the study and about their potential vulnerability as
research subjects.

For, to paraphrase George Bernard Shaw, medical researchers and their subjects are two groups separated by a common language. Whether you are reading Northfield's rosy press releases, PolyHeme's fawning media coverage, or the cloned PowerPoint slides screened in "community consultation" events from San Diego to Detroit, it quickly becomes clear that artful semantic fulcra have been employed to render the forcing of subjects into research ethically palatable. Like other apologists for investigative indenture, PolyHeme researchers tend to deploy medical jargon in a semantic sleight-of-hand that implies relationships and freedoms that do not exist.

Research subjects routinely are called "patients" in press releases, educational materials, and community meetings, which suggests a nonexistent doctor-patient relationship. The patient physician dyad, the traditional Western healing relationship, is based on a patient's unalloyed trust in his physician and the physician's strong sense of concern and responsibility toward her patient: a beautiful relationship, but it is not to be found here.

Were the PolyHeme recipients aware that the researcher was withholding from them the troubled medical history of HBOCs in general and PolyHeme in particular, were they aware that the researcher was paid a typical bounty of $10,000 per subject, and were they able to see that random ciphers on a computer-generated slip, rather than a doctor's clinical judgment, dictated the infusion liquid, the "patients" would have a better appreciation that no doctor-patient relationship reigns here. Similarly, PolyHeme is relentlessly referred to as a "treatment," and often as "safe" although neither its efficacy nor

72   its relative safety has been demonstrated: In fact, both are in serious question.

Jargon disguises the nature of transactions as well: People whose organs are taken without permission after death are referred to as "donors," which implies the appropriation was voluntary. Poor subjects who have been paid $4,000 to participate in malaria experiments are called "volunteers," and so are those who have no idea that they are being subjected to research.

During a university lecture I gave about ethically troubled medical research, an auditor criticized my use of the term "medical experiments" as "inflammatory." I was a bit surprised, given that I had limned the etymology of "experiment," including the definition given by Claude Bernard, author of *An Introduction to the Study of Experimental Medicine*, who wrote, "Experiment is fundamentally only induced observation." But I also remembered enough high-school Latin to shed some light on the discomfort. *Periculum*, "danger," is an inherent part of "experiment"—the word and the thing.

To experiment is to risk success or failure, and when human lives and health hang in the balance, the stakes are high indeed. It is true that terms such as "medical study" have come to be preferred, and for understandable reason: They now seem more benign. But these terms are not more accurate than "experiment" when the researcher manipulates variables and observes the effects on the bodies and minds of human subjects. Human medical experimentation is an accepted umbrella term for many of the more popular variants, so why does it provoke such wide discomfort?

After all, from the inception of modern ethical research assessments, "experimentation" was the default general term, wielded by investigators as well as by their critics. The first reference to human medical investigations, in the Nuremberg Code's first tenet, uses "experiment" twice when it reads in part "before the acceptance of an affirmative decision by the experimental subject, there should be made known to him the nature, duration, and purpose of the experiment."

The early authoritative classics of the field, from Henry K. Beecher's 1959 *Experimentation in Man* to his advisor Maurice Pappworth's 1967 *Human Guinea Pigs Here and Now: Experimentation on Man,* use the verboten word. The title of Jay Katz's seminal *Experimentation with Human Beings: The Authority of the Investigator, Subject, Professions, and State in the Human Experimentation Process,* like the Nuremberg Code, uses it twice.

Neither do respected works by research insiders shy from the term, such as *Who Goes First? The Story of Self-Experimentation in Medicine,* by Lawrence K. Altman, or *The Human Radiation Experiments* by the Advisory Committee on Human Radiation Experiments. As recently as 2015, Oxford Brookes professor Paul Weindling published his *Victims and Survivors of Nazi Human Experiments: Science and Suffering in the Holocaust.*

But by the time I began a public-health fellowship in 1992, the word "experimentation" was beginning to mutate. In fact, the fate of the word "mutation" itself provides a good parallel for the trajectory of "experiment" in the human-research context.

"Mutation," from the Latin verb *mutare,* to change, originally referred to tissue or genetic changes induced by radiation in a neutral or even benign manner, as when tumors shrunk after exposure: "mutation" was devoid of dread.

By 1911, however, more than fifty cases of X-ray-induced cancer had been reported in researchers who worked with

74   radioactive substances, followed by the ugly deaths of young
      "radium girls" who painted luminous watch dials with radium-
      226 and mesothorium. Such reports helped transform the
      public image of radiation and American scientists as willing
      to exploit radiation's injurious power for twisted curiosity or
      wealth. The word "mutation" now fills Americans with dread.

      Similarly, researchers now dislike "experiment," and not
      only because it reminds subjects of abuses, such as that of
      African Americans, prisoners, and Jews, but also of the danger,
      or *periculum,* inherent in even ethically conducted research.

      As Carl Elliott's "Whatever Happened to Human Exper-
      imentation?" points out, surveyed patients ranked the phrase
      "medical study" as the most benign, and "medical experiment"
      as so hazardous that some would risk joining one only if they
      were terminally ill. The term has been "purged," Elliott writes.

      The resulting newspeak, like other problematic linguistic
      choices discussed here, serves to reinforce the therapeutic illu-
      sion by masking the hazards of human studies. Words are pow-
      erful and word choices can limit researchers' ability to carry out
      the communication mandates upon which consent rests.

      In 1984, Orwell warns us, "The purpose of Newspeak was
      not only to provide a medium of expression for the worldview
      and mental habits proper to the devotees of INGSOC, but to
      make all other modes of thought impossible."

      In perhaps the most puzzling deployment of opaque jargon,
      some PolyHeme researchers invoke the ethical term "equi-
      poise" in speaking to laypersons. This term denotes a genuine
      uncertainty concerning the relative merits of treatments: Is
      the demonstrated standard of care, or the experimental sub-
      stance, in this case PolyHeme, superior? In order for research

to be ethical, the investigator is supposed to inhabit a genuine state of uncertainty about the tested modalities' relative merits: If she knew or strongly suspected that one treatment was better, she would be obligated to offer only that treatment to the subject. But an April 28, 2008, *JAMA* article unveiling the consistently poor performance of HBOCs calls this supposed uncertainty into serious question.

It is disturbing to reflect that as informed consent has been taken off the table, and with it, individual autonomy, thousands of people who share racial designations as Black and Hispanic are being addressed as if they are monolithic entities a single animus and no real right to say *yes* or *no*.

I was troubled by parallels to other sites where community consent is urged as a substitute for actual informed consent, notably in poor developing nations where researchers assure us that poor natives prefer the consent of a headman to individual informed consent. Sometimes this view is promulgated over the insistence of local physicians and ethicists who decry it as a cynical ploy to enroll poor Black and brown natives of developing countries without informed consent. At other times, as in Pfizer's 1996 trial of the experimental antibiotic Trovan in Kano, Nigeria, government-required consent and permission forms were forged or postdated after the study ended and eleven children died.

Despite the scant notification of many PolyHeme trial sites, two thousand people requested blue bracelets by March 2006, and at least eleven, including Martha, asked to be released from the trial once they learned what had been done to them.

Of course, they had already received PolyHeme, so they could not really be released: Only their data could be discarded.

Others may not have asked to be released because they understood there was no advantage in doing so. We do not know how many subjects took no action because they never knew that they had been infused with PolyHeme.

Northfield's stockholders were concerned about its lack of transparency and its free manner with data. The ANH trial results revealed that the subjects who received PolyHeme had a heart attack rate that was approximately 40 percent higher than those who had received saline. Accordingly, stockholders represented by Pomerantz, Haudek, Block, Grossman & Gross LLP commenced a class-action suit against the biotech on April 3, 2006. Considering the low present value of the company, any such suits may garner little.

But PolyHeme's human subjects may find justice just as elusive. The final data from the study's final (Phase III) trial showed that those subjects who received PolyHeme suffered a 3 percent heart-attack rate as opposed to only 1 percent in those who received saline. In May 2009, the FDA denied PolyHeme approval for use in humans because the study showed no clinical benefit and the safety data show that it placed patients at a higher risk of serious adverse events.

Martha says, "I was angry about being used without my permission, but I didn't know that PolyHeme was harming people until I read it in the newspaper. I called a lawyer right away, but he wouldn't help me. He said, 'You didn't die, so you have no case.'"

Northfield's stock share fell 51 percent and it ceased construction of the new complex it had been building to manufacture PolyHeme. On June 1, 2009, it announced that it had filed for bankruptcy. For months afterward, its website still referred to a "reorganization," but by June 2009, most new press reports I found concerned the shareholders' class-action suit.

However, the news media ignored medical victims like Martha who had survived, but with life-altering injuries. "I had suffered so much trauma. My whole body was open from my breast all the way down my torso. They performed a colostomy and they couldn't close me up for a long time. I returned to the hospital for several major surgeries, and the impact of the gunshot tore my retina, so I had to go in for eye surgery. My vision is pretty good now, I can see, but little waves make it seem as if something is always going across my field of vision.

"My body is disfigured now, There are a myriad of things wrong with me and I can't do half the things I used to do; I just have to accept that."

Perhaps the psychological scars are the worst. Martha still cannot sleep well, haunted by nightmares and fear despite the dog she bought for protection.

"But I'm walking. I'm able to live in my own home. I'm just glad to be alive and independent.

"But when I think of the research they did on me, I lose my peace of mind: How can they do that? How can they use you in an experiment without telling you what they want to do?"

In contravention to Martha's outrage, researchers have begun publishing reports using limited study data in an attempt to show that nonconsensual research does not violate research ethics, patient' rights, or preferentially affect communities of color. The reports are neither conclusive nor reassuring.

In 2019, survey results from a limited group of nonconsensual experiments were published in a *JAMA* article entitled

78   "Public Approval of Exception from Informed Consent in Emergency Clinical Trials." Among other things, it noted that the FDA has granted permission for more than forty Exception from Informed Consent, or EFIC, trials during the past two decades, and these trials have enrolled more than 45,000 patients, a very low estimate that doesn't include many large nonconsensual studies like the Department of Defense's anthrax vaccination program. African Americans made up 29.3 percent of a group of 17,302 survey participants, but they represented only 13.4 percent of the U.S. population in 2018, meaning that they were twice as likely to be conscripted into medical experimentation. Moreover, racial data were available for only 72 percent of returned surveyed participants, so the number of African Americans could be much higher.

Still, this article purports to tell us how the public views legalized nonconsensual research. The survey looks at 42,448 responses from twenty-seven such studies conducted between 1996 and October 2017 and assures the reader that, "All trials granted an EFIC must submit documentation of compliance with EFIC regulations to a publicly available docket at the FDA." But as we have seen, violations of the conditions imposed on nonconsensual research are common, from failure to notify the greater community that the research was underway to withholding consent from the conscious to withholding the standard of care once it is available in hospitals to violating a state's Patient's Bill of Rights, as occurred in North Carolina.

The report goes on to claim that "58.4 percent approved of EFIC in *principle*, 68.6 percent approved of *family-member enrollment*, 73.0 percent approved of *personal enrollment*, and

86.5 percent approved of *community inclusion.*" We need a definition of the italicized terms to know what this means. But no matter how they are defined, the percentages are far too low to justify claiming popular support. Medical ethicist Robert Veatch has written that claims of endorsement by the public would have to prove two things: that community members approve of 1) the study itself and 2) of administering it without getting the consent of or even informing subjects. He also indicated that one cannot claim a mandate for nonconsensual study exists unless about 95 percent of those affected approve. Even the rosiest assessment reported in this survey hovered at about 70 percent.

Even worse, a survey disclaimer gives one pause: "Groups surveyed with higher proportions of *African American and male respondents had lower rates of EFIC approval, and these groups were underrepresented in surveys relative to their enrollment in EFIC trials.*" Because African Americans are underrepresented in these surveys, they convey no reliable information about their acceptance of nonconsensual studies. It is telling that the paper doesn't offer the exact rates for African Americans' approval. The failure to quantify it immediately after the recounting of specific figures for approval by the majority populations leads one to wonder just how much lower it was—15 percent lower? 90 percent lower?

Other largescale studies consistently find that the majority of African Americans, who are disproportionate subjects in such trials, are less likely to approve of such research.

A survey conducted by Michele Goodwin, Chancellor's Professor of Law at the University of California at Irvine and the

80   author of *Black Markets: The Supply and Demand of Human Body Parts,* also revealed that 80 percent of African Americans surveyed reject presumed consent as an unacceptable method for procuring tissues.

History helps to explain this aversion.

Today, using residents from the minority-group catchment in nonconsensual "EFIC" studies maintains disproportionately African American areas in investigational servitude.

"The Other"

The Nuremberg Code is the most important influence on U.S. law governing human medical research, but as we've seen, it was quickly diluted in the interests of researcher convenience. This forced many Americans into studies that violated their right to consent.

In 1941, before the Nuremberg Code was adopted, President Franklin Roosevelt established the Office of Scientific Research, which governed the Committee on Medical Research (CMR). It focused on ameliorating medical problems faced by American soldiers. Under its aegis, the U.S. began surreptitiously testing weaponized disease on unsuspecting Americans. A vaccine against dysentery, which the CMR feared might decimate U.S. troops, was forced on the intellectually disabled, revealing side effects and deaths that proved it too toxic for military use. Intellectually disabled patients in Pennhurst, Pennsylvania, and at Ypsilanti State Hospital, Michigan, were also used to test anti-influenza preparations.

As often happens, the ethical argument of utilitarianism was invoked, which is British philosopher Jeremy Bentham's exhortation to choose that course that provides "the greatest good for the greatest number of people." This consequentialist approach allows the sacrifice of the autonomy and welfare of the few for the majority. A profound flaw in utilitarian schemes is that "the few" are too often also the powerless and the marginalized, such as African Americans, the poor, children, or the intellectually disabled. The tyranny of the majority is used to sacrifice the marginalized for the welfare of the valorized majority. Invoking utilitarianism supported decades of government-sponsored, often military, research that violates human dignity.

Dark Compulsion

For example, informed consent, and even simple consent, have been withheld consistently in research with African Americans.

The frequent claim that this group has rarely been included in medical research sounds plausible only because historians of medicine have typically ignored the African American experience. For centuries, Black Americans have been coerced into a multitude of nontherapeutic, dangerous, and abusive medical experiments. *Medical Apartheid: The Dark History of Medical Experimentation on Black Americans from Colonial Times to the Present* recounts how mythology about their "subhuman" bodies and minds combined with a legal system of chattel enslavement to rob Black Americans of bodily ownership and autonomy.

Whether subjected to laissez-faire experimentation on the plantation, early clinics, or other institutions, Black Americans were sold to doctors expressly for nineteenth-century research and physician-training purposes.

On October 12, 1838, for example a Dr. T. Stillman placed an advertisement in the *Charleston Mercury*: "Wanted: FIFTY NEGROES. Any person having sick negroes, considered incurable by their respective physicians and wishing to dispose of them . . . the highest cash prize will be paid upon application as above."

Every important reproductive surgery advance was tested on Black women because, unlike white women, they could not say *no*. In Alabama, James Marion Sims, the Victorian "father of American gynecology," forced Black women he held captive in a shack on his property to undergo repeated experimental genital surgeries over the course of five years. Historian Walter Fisher sums it up: "It is most improbable that Sims and [his assistant] Bozeman could have established so remarkable a surgical schedule without the slave system which provided the experimental subjects."

Sims also used a shoemaker's awl to the pry open the skulls of Black newborn infants in an experimental technique to address neonatal tetany. He had his medical students tie a recalcitrant slave named Sam to a barber's chair in order to force upon him new experimental techniques as he removed his lower jaw.

The infamous "Tuskegee syphilis study," conducted by the U.S. Public Health Service between 1932 and 1972 used approximately six hundred Black men who had been diagnosed with syphilis. They were not treated but were maintained in an infected state, tracked, studied, and ultimately autopsied because researchers wished to document what they claimed was

84   a disparate disease course in Blacks. The PHS sought to prove
      that Blacks were spared the neurological devastation of the
      final "tertiary stage" of syphilis because their brains and ner-
      vous systems were less complex than those of whites. The men
      in the study were never informed that they were being used as
      research subjects.

      African Americans were forced into experimentation in
      every arena of U.S. medicine—eugenics, surgery, anatomical
      display, cognitive and psychological disorders, infectious dis-
      eases, radiation, pediatrics, and inmates of the carceral state—
      as were Hispanics, some other minorities, and the poor. Their
      investigative servitude didn't end with enslavement nor even
      with de jure segregation.

      More recent twentieth- and twenty-first-century abuses
      include the enrollment of Black women into the Medical Uni-
      versity of South Carolina in Charleston's narcotic-treatment
      research without their knowledge in 1994. When these preg-
      nant women presented themselves to the prenatal clinic for
      assistance in combating their drug problems, the university
      turned them over to the police, then enrolled them in drug
      studies without their knowledge.

      In 1989, a banned experimental vaccine with a his-
      tory of adverse effects was tested on mostly Black and His-
      panic Los Angeles children without their parents' consent. And
      from 1994 to 1996, New York City boys, all younger brothers of
      delinquents and identified via law enforcement officials, were
      enrolled without voluntary consent in experiments that tried
      to determine whether there was a genetic connection to vio-
      lent or antisocial behavior, by giving them the cardiotoxic diet

drug fenfluramine, which is now banned. Law enforcement officials illegally helped researchers to coerce Black parents into
bringing their children into the dangerous study.

In 2001, Baltimore's Johns Hopkins–affiliated Kennedy
Krieger Institute was found guilty by a Maryland appellate court
of encouraging unwitting Black families with small children to
move into lead-contaminated housing as part of a study into the
cheapest way to abate indoor lead levels. The children's changing
blood lead levels were tested to evaluate the degree of abatement,
leading the court to call them "canaries in the coal mine."

Of course, the scourge of coercion was not at all confined to
racial minorities.

Radiating Coercion

One of the most disturbing human studies was done at the University of Chicago, where 102 unwitting subjects at state schools
were fed the radioactive elements strontium and cesium. The
Quaker Oats Company even supported a study at the Fernald
School in Waltham, Massachusetts, where thirty orphans were
given radioactive oatmeal in a program sponsored by the AEC.
Upper-class children were not spared experimental coercion
as when incoming students at Ivy League universities were
forced to submit to the taking of nude photos as part of eugenics
research. Medical and science students who participated in
research projects have done so in part because of tacit or overt
pressure to cooperate in their professors' research agenda.

Between the 1945 bombing of Hiroshima and July 1947, the
scientists of the Manhattan Project followed the construction
of the bomb with a chilling second act: medical experimentation

86   on hundreds of unsuspecting Americans. In one such program, soldiers were shipped to the desert for deliberate exposure to nuclear detonations. In another, unsuspecting patients in private and public hospitals—from Strong Memorial Hospital in Rochester, New York, to Vanderbilt University Hospital's prenatal clinic in Nashville—were injected with plutonium infused with fluorine or were otherwise used as subjects in various experiments to calibrate the physical damage associated with various dosages of radioactive matter.

Eileen Welsome's *The Plutonium Files* detailed the nationwide experiment in which Americans from all walks of life were secretly injected with radioactive plutonium by doctors at medical institutions under contract to the Atomic Energy Commission. Military physician Joseph Howland injected Ebb Cade with 4.7 micrograms—forty-one times the normal lifetime exposure—of plutonium, "the most dangerous chemical known," according to Col. Stafford Warren, director of the Manhattan Project's Medical Section.

This never should have happened, because in late 1946, the Judicial Council of the American Medical Association had set new, widely disseminated standards for the protection of human subjects, establishing that three requirements must be satisfied: (1) the voluntary consent of the person on whom the experiment is to be performed, (2) the danger of each experiment must be previously investigated by animal experimentation, and (3) the experiment must be performed under proper medical protection and management.

Despite the new rule, government scientists justified these radiation studies, for which President Bill Clinton apologized in 1995. Clinton said that the experiments were essential to

protect American soldiers who could be exposed to radiation
by the Soviet Union. But as AEC physician Shields Warren
observed in 1950, "It's not long since we got through trying Germans for doing exactly the same thing."

Lawrence Altman's *Who Goes First? The Story of Self-Experimentation in Medicine* documents doctors who followed
a long tradition of first following animal studies with limited
self-experimentation by testing substances or procedures on
themselves before experimenting with appreciable numbers of
human subjects. Testing themselves first was a symbolic act, a
claim that the measures were not inordinately harmful, and also
a signal that they were willing to risk their lives in the name of
science.

But the radiation researchers of the 1940s refused to experiment on themselves. "We considered doing such experiments
at one time," Wright Langham said. "But plutonium is considered to be sufficiently potentially dangerous to discourage our
doing absorption experiments upon ourselves."

Even researchers who questioned the moral acceptability of
doing nonconsensual studies acquiesced, in part because they
had been conditioned to accept authority blindly, as Yale psychology professor Stanley Milgram's classic 1963 experiment,
"Obedience to Authority," illustrates.

During this experiment, most students obeyed a researcher's orders to inflict increasingly powerful electric shocks to
an unseen, screaming subject, which helped to illuminate the
mindset under which nascent researchers fail to protest or cease
conducting questionable, even abusive, experiments despite
their ethical qualms. More than 80 percent of the participants kept going after delivering up to 150 volts. Shockingly, 65

88   percent of them kept going until they reached 450 volts, even
     though the unseen subjects' screams were replaced by a silence
     that suggested the subject was no longer able to respond, having
     been rendered unconscious—or worse. Unbeknownst to the
     students, the shocks were not real and the "subjects" were actors.

     "Its conclusion," according to the *New York Times*, "was
     that most ordinary people were willing to administer what they
     believed to be painful, even dangerous, electric shocks to inno-
     cent people if a man in a white lab coat told them to." Unfor-
     tunately, little seems to have changed: In 2008, Jerry Burger of
     Santa Clara University replicated the experiment. His findings,
     published in *American Psychologist*, are nearly identical to Mil-
     gram's: Seven of ten students administered the highest-potency
     shock.

     ## Caged Subjects

     Like enslavement, research with the incarcerated "was a remark-
     able experimental system that blurred the lines between punish-
     ment and research, " writes Nathaniel Comfort, a professor in the
     Johns Hopkins University Institute of the History of Medicine.

     In the wake of Nuremberg, U.S. prisoners have been burned,
     had cancerous cells implanted into their bodies, have been sub-
     jected to damaging radiation including on their genitals and
     corneas, and been forced to undergo experimental lobotomies.

     Researchers have long been comfortable with using the
     bodies and minds of prisoners for dangerous research. Robert
     Boyle, the seventeenth-century father of chemistry, pro-
     posed, "Trayal might be made on some genuine human bodies,
     especially those of Malefactors." Inmates have often been the
     first group that doctors turn to for experiments, from testing

vaccines to using cadavers for dissection. *The Journal of the National Medical Association* proposed in 1910 that prisoners were the most appropriate medical research subjects, and that criminals could pay off their debt to society by being tested upon, even if they were unwilling and unwitting.

Throughout the twentieth century, the supposedly "free consent" of American prisoners was circumscribed in several ways. In the most extreme cases, prisoners' right to say *no* simply did not exist. Between January 1967 and April 1968, imprisoned subjects at the California Medical Facility were given succinylcholine, also known as Anectine, a neuromuscular compound that paralyzed muscles so that the prisoner could not move—or breathe. Many likened the terrifying experience to drowning in fetters. When five of the sixty-four selected prisoners refused to participate in the experiment, the institution's Special Treatment Board gave permission on behalf of the recalcitrant men for them to be injected against their will.

But prison administrations usually exerted subtler pressure, in the form of authority figures and even prisoner advocates such as social workers, who steered penniless inmates to research studies. Nick DiSpoldo, an inmate in the Arizona State Prison, told the *New York Times*› that parole boards routinely held a refusal to participate in research against inmates seeking release.

Plenty of evidence exists suggesting that coercion is indeed a key element whenever supposed consent was given by prisoners. Clinical medical ethicists today tend to define *coercion* narrowly and without much precision, so many would argue that the inmates may have been induced but not coerced. Such opinions fail to take into account the coercive features of the dangerous prison environment. The hell of prison life made the research laboratory, feared and abhorred by many on the outside, an irresistible haven.

Moreover, the pay for becoming a research subject was far greater than typical jobs in the prison kitchen or laundry, and money had a very different meaning for inmates than it had for outsiders. Inmates sought not only commissary baubles and delicacies to brighten life but, more important, the price of freedom—or, at least, of safety.

Jails are full of people, both guilty and innocent, who are there only because they are too poor to make bail. Between the 1940s and 1970s, bail bondsmen typically would spring an inmate for a down payment of 10 percent of his bail, so that a man jailed in lieu of a $500 bond could buy his freedom within weeks with the $50 he earned from a single medical experiment.

Several inmates also mention a motivation about which the news media kept silent: The human landscape of prison is largely devoid of affection, and incarcerated men described time in the research laboratory as a respite for the psyche, a place where one could go for a while to be addressed and touched with kindness, dignity, and concern.

Some researchers exploited this to psychologically manipulate the prisoners, undercutting the ability to give truly voluntary consent. Alfred Kligman, who conducted abusive research throughout the Pennsylvania's Stygian Holmesburg prison system for decades, said:

> Many of the prisoners for the first time in their lives find themselves in the role of important human beings. We say to them "You're important: We need you." Once this is

established these guys will knock their brains out to please you. If the experiment does not pan out, they get depressed. They become emotionally involved with the project. The capacity to respond to love is greater than most people realize. I feel almost like a scoundrel—like Machiavelli—because of what I can do to them.

In the 1970s, widely publicized abuses, deaths, and violations of informed consent in U.S. prisons fueled legislation to ban most types of prison research except those that could be shown to help prisoners themselves. But in 2006, an Institute of Medicine panel, whose decisions are usually adopted into law, recommended that prisons be reopened to wider research.

Why? Today, prisoners make ideal subjects in Phase I experiments, where being able to standardize some elements of subjects' living conditions and track subjects over time without them being "lost to follow up" is critical. Phase I refers to the first phase in clinical trials, in which a potential drug's safety is tested, typically by giving it to healthy subjects and studying any side effects or adverse effects after its administration. Phase II trials aim at determining dosing requirements and demonstrating therapeutic efficacy. Phase III trials are on a larger scale and usually compare a drug's results with standard treatments.

Have the abuses recurred? It's hard to tell, because the closed nature of prisons facilitates the shrouding of abuses and even violations of the law. The prevalence of for-profit medical caregiving in prisons encourages a profitable crisis-oriented mode of healthcare provision that discourages monitoring and surveillance.

92   **Laboratory of the West?**

The failure to elicit consent is not confined to the United States. Most U.S. corporate medical studies are now carried out by U.S. research institutions abroad, usually in developing-world sites where trials can be conducted far more cheaply and rapidly than in the U.S.

But eliciting consent from marginalized populations abroad, although legally required, is rarely monitored, more rarely enforced, and has never been a popular move among researchers. In 1964, Harvard researcher Dr. Francis D. Moore wrote:

> Several years ago an individual from this country went to Nigeria to try out a new measles vaccine on a lot of small children. Now how exactly are you going to explain to a Black African jungle mother the fact that measles vaccine occasionally produces encephalitis but that more important than that it might sensitize the child for the rest of his life to some other protein in the vaccine? . . . Can you imagine trying to explain that to a jungle mother? . . . One of the greatest assets of a good doctor is the ability to look a patient in the eye and have the patient go along with him on a hazardous course of treatment. . . . The same quality is exhibited by a medical experimenter when he looks at [a] patient and says that he thinks everything is all right.

In 2000, a cancer researcher at South Africa's Witwatersrand University named Werner Bezwoda was fired after giving extremely high doses of chemotherapy to Black breast-cancer patients without obtaining informed consent. And an America doctor, Michael Swango, was convicted of murder after pleading guilty to killing three American patients with injections of potassium, but he is also suspected of killing as many as sixty other patients during the 1980s and 1990s, mostly in Zimbabwe and Zambia.

Also in Zimbabwe, a Scottish anesthesiologist named Richard McGown was accused of five murders and convicted in 1995 of killing two infants by injecting them with morphine. Wouter Basson, the former head of Project Coast, South Africa's chemical and biological weapons unit under apartheid, oversaw a malicious nationwide research agenda that included experiments aimed at creating agents to selectively harm or sterilize black Africans in the guise of vaccines. He was charged with killing hundreds of Black South Africans and Namibians from 1979 to 1987, many via injected poisons.

Today, 80 percent of U.S. clinical trials use subjects in the developing world, especially the global South where high-quality research can be conducted quickly and cheaply. Recent laws have mandated including some U.S. subjects in these trials as well, but only 25 percent must be U.S. subjects and oversight of this is rare: So, it seems, is compliance. In countries where subjects enjoy little access to healthcare, they are told they are being "treated" and are often unaware that the "treatments" are experimental modalities and are part of medical research.

For example, as mentioned previously, drug giant Pfizer paid $75 million in 2011 to settle claims that children in Kano state, Nigeria, were harmed or even killed after they were given an experimental drug, Trovan, during a meningitis epidemic. Nigerian parents protested and stormed courts in Kano and Manhattan.

94   **Presumed Consent**

Another aspect of foreign medicine that catalyzed today's assault on informed consent: presumed consent. In some European countries, such as Spain and Greece, organ donors cannot withhold permission to retrieve their organs after death. One still needs to procure permission for drug testing and much research, but involuntary collection reigns for organ donation. If you are brain-dead or dead, your organs will be collected and distributed without your consent. Some European nations provide legal routes to opting out by you or your survivors if you express a refusal to donate, but others do not.

What those who urge the U.S. to adopt such research schemes fail to appreciate is that they seldom travel well. They are often practiced within cultures very different from ours with superior single payer healthcare that leads to equitable access, lesser ethnic friction (sometimes), and higher levels of trust based on histories that are not marked, as the U.S. is, by dramatic examples of bias and inequitable treatment. Spain, for example, maintains not only presumed consent but also some ambulances whose role is not to speed to the ailing and save their lives, but to retrieve viable organs immediately from those declared dead at the scene. But when New York City attempted to pioneer a similar program around 2008—the "organ recovery ambulance" under the Rapid Organ Recovery service—widespread outrage ensued and the program never got off the ground.

Heartened by U.S. transplantation advocates who urge the adoption of presumed consent for procuring organs, U.S. advocates of exception from informed consent (EFIC) research point to presumed consent as a model for compelling human medical experimentation.

Presumed consent advocates point to the insufficiency of organs freed up by voluntary donation and insist that involuntary donation—presumed consent—will free up much-needed organs and save lives. Curiously, their arguments cling to the illogical nomenclature of "donors" and "donation." This not only veils the fact that these organs are being conscripted, but that an unacknowledged market for organs exists in the U.S., as described in Michele Bratcher Goodwin's book *Black Markets: The Supply and Demand of Body Parts.* Advocates also insist that no major religions proscribe organ transplantation. They seemingly are comfortable with proscription by "minor" or unrecognized religions—and by individuals' beliefs that may not rely upon the precepts of organized religion.

This belief that presumed consent is a powerful tool to bridge the "organ gap" sounds plausible, but it is not necessarily borne out by the empirical evidence, as experts in England learned when they contemplated adopting presumed consent. Consider that some presumed-consent countries like Spain and Croatia have high donor rates (each boasts 40.2 donors per million inhabitants), but others, like Greece, maintain low rates of only 6 donors per million people.

This is because presumed consent alone doesn't drive the variation in organ donation rates. Infrastructure, organizational schemes, wealth, investment in healthcare, availability of donors, public attitudes, and culture all play murkily understood roles. This led a 2009 report by England's Technology Assessment Programme to conclude, "It cannot be inferred from this that the introduction of presumed consent legislation per se leads to an increase in donation rates."

96 Presumed Consent at Home

Presumed consent is a policy in the U.S., too, but it is a well-hidden one. Some cities in most U.S. states have "medical examiners' laws," which cite conditions under which the medical examiner can appropriate tissues, organs, and entire cadavers for research as well as for transplantation. No permission is required of the "donor" or his family and families sometimes complain that their loved ones' bodies have been withheld from them and organs removed without notification.

This helps to explain why a slew of earlier surveys revealed animosity toward constructs like "presumed consent," which in the U.S. refers to the failure to elicit permission when obtaining organs for transplantation because researchers "presume" that the "donors" would agree to surrender them.

"African Americans presume not to consent," said Clive O. Callender, chief of transplant surgery at Howard University. He is the founder of the Minority Organ and Tissue Transplantation and Education Program and the highest-profile proponent of African-American organ and tissue donation in the nation. African Americans have responded generously to pleas for organ donation: the success of programs such as MOTTEP gives testimony to that. But presumed consent is anathema to this group. "There are specific reasons why we are often suspicious of attempts to part us from our organs," Callender said, citing the long history of African-American body appropriation and high contemporary rates of amputation.

Today, 80 percent of African Americans live in urban areas and, proportionally, five African Americans die in accidents for every four whites, high rates that increase the risk for compulsion into EFIC studies. Because the homicide rate is eight to ten times higher among African Americans, Black bodies are also more likely than others to end up in a milieu where they fall prey to presumed consent.

Callender is not the only scholar who has quantified African-American opposition to presumed consent. A survey conducted by Goodwin also revealed that 80 percent of African Americans surveyed reject presumed consent as an unacceptable method for procuring tissues.

History helps to explain this aversion. Medical experiments often draw subjects from an institution's "catchment area"—typically, that community surrounding it. Many medical institutions are located in predominately African-American and poverty-stricken areas. As I explain in *Medical Apartheid*, this is not accidental but by design. The proximity of Black bodies for display, teaching, practice, and training material was an economic boon for medical schools and a selling point in recruiting medical students. African-American patients were subjected to research as "repayment" for treatment in subterranean reduced-price charity clinics—even though no amount of money could buy a Black patient a bed in a private ward.

Even after death, these bodies served pedagogical purposes as they were similarly appropriated for anatomical dissection. This was as true in the North of the U.S. as in the South, but enslavement, and later, de jure racial segregation, reinforced the appropriation of Black bodies. Today, using residents from the catchment in nonconsensual "EFIC" studies restores these people, who remain disproportionately African American, to investigational servitude.

98   Conflating "emergency treatment" with often-profitable medical experimentation and invoking presumed consent are not the only arguments for dispensing with consent for medical research.

Researchers also invoke utilitarianism, insisting that just as the right of individuals to control the fate of their organs after death is outweighed by the greater benefit to the many, the putative benefits of research outweigh an individual's right to say *yes* or *no* to medical research. Some researchers also question the judgment of patients who may "erroneously" decide against becoming research subjects because (in the opinion of the researchers) they are ill-informed, confused, or irrationally fearful.

Still others invoke an individual's moral responsibility to participate in research. Russ Gruen, MD, Professor of Surgery in Singapore's Lee Kong Chian School of Medicine, indicts as "morally weak" the argument of those who say, in essence, "I'm prepared to benefit from medical research, but I'm not prepared to be counted on to help others in the future."

The U.S. history of medicine has been curated to obscure the nature of questionable or exploitative treatment of its marginalized populations. Semantics have also been recruited in a manner that robs the complaints of the powerless of credibility. Nowhere has this exculpatory semantics been practiced so dramatically as in the long practice of disguising subjects as "patients" and experimental ventures as "treatments." Apologists for questionable research also sometimes ascribe objections and fears to "paranoia" and a belief in "conspiracy theories" instead of discounting them with facts.

Some claim that the rich U.S. matrix of laws, including those subsumed under the Code of Federal Regulations, protects research subjects, but such laws mean little when they are unmonitored, unenforced, or so vaguely worded as to be meaningless. In 2011, for example, the Presidential Bioethics Commission issued a report on protecting human research subjects entitled *Moral Science*. It made much of the U.S.'s "robust" protections—the very rules that permit and legitimize the breaches of informed consent discussed here.

Moreover, many laws govern only federally funded research. The Department of Health and Human Services' Office for Human Research Protections has jurisdiction only over research funded by the department, and few people realize how little oversight the government offers to protect the subjects of privately sponsored studies. The FDA oversees drug and biologicals safety, but it inspects only 1 percent of all clinical trials. Moreover, a 2007 HHS report revealed that it conducts "more inspections that verify clinical trial data than inspections that focus on human-subject protections."

In fact, it was not until 2005, Carl Elliott points out, that FDA inspectors were even given a code number that would enable them to report a study's "failure to protect the rights, safety, and welfare of subjects."

Cold-Blooded Killer

Storms, blizzards, ill-fated hiking excursions, snowmobile accidents, and car breakdowns in frigid weather all make hypothermia a familiar enemy in many hospital emergency departments.

Hypothermia is a medical emergency caused when cold exposure drives the core body temperature below 95°F. As the body temperature falls, brain function decreases, replacing shivering and hunger with nausea, lethargy, slurred speech, and confusion. Instead of seeking warmth, apathy sets in, and some hypothermics remove their clothing before falling into a sleep that progresses to coma. As the body's core temperature falls below 82.4°F, abnormal electrical rhythms develop, including ventricular fibrillation in which the heart fails to pump blood. This deadly cardiac arrest may also occur during medical treatment when the hypothermic person's body is rewarmed. Brain activity slows dramatically as the pupils dilate, and the victim appears comatose or dead.

When the core temperature plummets to 68°F, brain function ceases, and at 50°F, the patient has crossed over into profound hypothermia. This dire state carries a mortality rate of around 40 percent, even with prompt attention within a Level 1 trauma center, wherein a patient can expect state-of-the-art emergency care.

The Triad of Death

Hypothermia is part of what doctors call "the triad of death" (falling blood-plasma pH and blood's inability to coagulate constitute the other deadly events). These events make a patient's resuscitation increasingly unlikely.

Like other deadly crises, hypothermia triggers the grim, controlled urgency of the emergency department as each team member slides into their role, uttering terse updates as the energetic rewarming, treating, and close monitoring of the patient, who faces a lingering threat of cardiac arrest until the crisis is resolved, takes effect, for good or ill.

In 2010, a study was published where Baltimore researchers, instead of treating victims' wounds with the standard of care, intentionally induced hypothermia in unwitting Black men who had suffered gunshot wounds. The researchers, led by Samuel Tisherman at the University of Maryland's R. Adams Cowley Shock Trauma Center, said they sought to discover whether the typically-fatal cold might help these men to survive their injuries. The study's formal name is Body Cooling Study: Emergency Preservation and Resuscitation for Cardiac Arrest from Trauma, or EPR-CAT.

Tisherman's team acknowledged that hypothermia is frequently fatal, but rationalized their acts by noting that a very small number of people, notably some infants, have survived drowning in cold water, although often with lingering health problems. Researchers wondered whether the slowed metabolism caused by hypothermia might be a protective factor.

The researchers were testing this in adults without asking their consent because, they explained, the subjects would be unconscious and unable to give it, and it meets the federal conditions for nonconsensual research under 21 CFR 50.23-4. However, there's no mention of how meeting the required conditions would be individually assessed, nor what provisions for consent would be made if a victim became conscious, as Martha Milete did during her PolyHeme infusion.

Why target Black men? A 2016 article in the *New Yorker* vaguely implies that it is because they suffer high rates of firearms deaths:

> Baltimore has one of the nation's highest rates of gun violence, and Shock Trauma admits at least two or three shooting victims each week—often, like Brandon Littlejohn, young Black men.

If Black men were the most frequent victims of death by gunfire and therefore gunfire posed a uniquely high risk to them, the Baltimore researchers might be able to construct a case that singling them out as subjects constitutes an equitable distribution of research risks and benefits. However, the U.S. leads the world in gun deaths, and most of these deaths are in white men: nine thousand white men died from firearms in 2012, compared to six thousand Black men. Moreover, in Baltimore in 2016, unarmed Black Americans were five times as likely as unarmed white Americans to be shot and killed by a police officer. Targeting of this marginalized racial minority is both unethical and illogical.

Being the most frequent victims of gunshot wounds is not an acceptable reason for subjecting a population to dangerous and involuntary experimental hypothermia, but if it were, that population would be white men.

Moreover, Black men suffer higher-than-normal rates from almost every form of heart disease, including congestive heart failure and heart attacks. In America, 44 percent of Black men suffer some form of heart disease, largely attributable to diabetes, hypertension, and obesity, but are not treated as successfully as are white men. True beneficence would entail addressing these verified disparate risks, so why single out for attention gun deaths, which not only affect mostly white men, but also play into an empathy-damping stereotype of Black male violence?

To justify inducing hypothermia, researchers claimed that the deadly condition offers a better chance for survival than the standard of care, which saves only about 5 percent of victims. But no data are offered to support this increased-survival claim, and the available evidence shows that not one person has been saved in this research with deadly hypothermia. In 2016, Tisherman indicated that the study results would be published within two years, but they were not. In 2020, university media officer Lisa Clough admitted that they still have not been published four years later, so we can't know how subjects have fared or whether *any* hypothermic subjects survived.

Tisherman did not respond to my repeated email and telephone requests to discuss this work, which were made both directly to him and through his university's media office. However, he did speak with a *New Scientist* reporter to whom he optimistically described the research not as a risky nonconsensual induction of hypothermia, but as cutting-edge "suspended animation" that his team hopes will buy patients time to recover.

But these are involuntary research subjects, not patients, and the term "suspended animation" is misleading because it implies that the hypothermia's effects are controllable and known to be reversible: They are not.

The intentional induction of hypothermia is presented as offering benefit to those forced into the experiment, but what we know about this medical crisis argues otherwise, especially when the *New Yorker* revealed that the 50°F *profound hypothermia*—with its 40 percent mortality rate—is precisely what researchers plan to induce in these young men. Touting the potential beneficence of inducing the deadliest-level hypothermia as cutting-edge experimental trauma "treatment" is an illogical inversion, but not an unusual one.

This rhetoric highlights the danger of encouraging research subjects to think of themselves as "patients." Such language leads the lay audience to suppose that their best health outcome is the goal of the "treatment," which is not the case in research. It implies that the efficacy and safety of an experimental approach, even one best known as part of the "triad of death," have been demonstrated: They have not.

The late Jay Katz had a name for this erroneous belief that an experimental subject will enjoy the rights accruing to patient. He called this the "therapeutic illusion." In 1996, shortly after the adoption of the CFR 21 50.24 exception to informed consent, he criticized the legalization of such research by warning against couching experimental drugs and techniques as "cutting-edge therapy" and implying that untested modalities are "treatment." He wrote:

One of my most fundamental objections to the regulation is this: that in its emphasis on therapeutic benefits, the FDA obscures the fact that some of the permissible research activities either hold out no promise for therapeutic benefit or are so vaguely defined that potential therapeutic benefit can be inferred when research is the predominant intent. Research is not treatment, and whenever clear distinctions are not made between the two, the waiver of informed consent becomes problematic because some human subjects are being recruited to serve the ends of others.

Nicola Twilley, author of the *New Yorker* article, expressed her concern that targeted African Americans subjects would object because they are fearful of medical research in general and distrustful because of "past abuses" such as the infamous 1932–1972 Tuskegee study.

"The Tuskegee study," which was actually conducted by the U.S. Public Health Service, not the university, is often inappropriately invoked by those without knowledge of the actual history of African Americans' abuse in the medical research arena, perhaps because it is the only abusive study they know of. But centuries of well-documented medical abuse and exploitation—not one infamous study—have encouraged a logical distrust in U.S. medical research. Moreover, as experts, including Matthew Wynia, MD, director of the Center for Bioethics and Humanities at the University of Colorado's Anschutz Medical Campus, has pointed out, it is not just African American wariness, but also the untrustworthiness of the U.S. medical system that has maintained this climate of fear.

Discussing one without the other pathologizes African Americans' logical reaction to centuries of abuse, past and present. Furthermore, Professor Thomas LaVeist's research at Johns Hopkins School of Public Health reveals that African Americans who had never heard of the Tuskegee study are more likely to fear medical experimentation than those who had, summarizing, "Our results cast doubt on the proposition that the widely documented race difference in mistrust of medical care results from the Tuskegee study. Rather, race differences in mistrust likely stem from broader historical and personal experiences."

The ethical abuse that should concern us in Tisherman's study is violation of *distributive justice*: Targeting African American men creates a situation in which they bear the deadly risks of the research, but stand to benefit least, because of their reduced access to healthcare in general and to cardiac technology in particular. The *New Yorker* and *New Scientist* remained silent on such ethical failures that would give the experiment proper context.

They also failed to discuss the hypothermia experiment in the context of a slew of other similar nonconsensual research studies such as those under the aegis of the massive Resuscitation Outcomes Consortium, or ROC, studies, which include a legion of other involuntary experiments, including infusion with heated saline and concentrated salt solutions.

Despite the glaring racial issues, this denial of consent and the attendant risks are not confined to people of color. It's important to remember that, thanks to function creep, involuntarily subjecting subjects to hypothermia for research purposes is a universal risk that would almost certainly extend to Americans of all ethnicities and other socioeconomic strata.

Other aspects of the *New Yorker* article are similarly devoid of context and reveal a profound naivete about nonconsensual-research practices. For example, allowing people to opt out of no-consent studies by wearing a special plastic "refusal" bracelet is a tactic that has been used since at least 2005 in various studies like that of PolyHeme and in the massive contemporary Resuscitation Outcomes Consortium. But the article intimates that it is Tisherman's invention:

> He designed a red rubber bracelet, in the style of Lance Armstrong's Livestrong wristbands, that says "No to EPR-CAT." (EPR-CAT is the trial's full name; *CAT* stands for *cardiac arrest from trauma.*)

The *New Yorker* article never mentions the troubled history of "no-consent" studies, their frequent violation of the federal law that mandates them, the increased death and debility that resulted from many of them, or the criticism of "community notification" as a poor substitute for informed consent.

Neither is the criticism from medical ethicists like Jay Katz mentioned as the article breezily dismisses the fact that in the community meeting, young Black men—the targeted subjects of this no-consent study—voiced their opposition, to no avail. Twilley writes:

> *Only two people* [italics mine] voiced objections: Both were young Black men, and both left before Tisherman could

speak to them. The first pointed at Tisherman, smiled, and said, "Y'all heard me say no." The second man, listening while Tisherman explained EPR to two women, announced, "We're guinea pigs—your body language says it!"

"Body Cooling Study," an online description of the study by the university, reads, "Once enrolled, patients can withdraw from the study at any time" but doesn't explain this claim. It seems fictitious, because not only have the unconscious subjects (*not* "patients") never been informed that they are in a study, and so they are unable to voice an objection. Moreover, once infused with cooling liquid without their permission, that risky procedure cannot be undone even in the unlikely event that they recover.

Had Tisherman agreed to speak with me, I also would have asked him not only whether any subjects had survived, but also about the fact that he will profit financially if his study findings are positive.

According to a note on the study's online description:

The principal investigator, Samuel Tisherman, MD, has *a financial interest in intellectual property for the development of the EPR procedure and some of the associated hardware including special catheters and accessories which have been licensed to EPR Technologies* [italics mine]. This means that it is possible that the results of this study could lead to personal profit for the individual investigator.

Tisherman's financial stake in the study's successful outcome creates a financial conflict of interest that makes its

results untrustworthy. Analyses consistently demonstrate that
medical-research results tend to emerge in concert with their
commercial backers' financial interests.

This conflict of interest also reveals how rarely the incentives
of medical researchers become part of the risk-benefit discussions. Rationales for conducting research focus on the puta
tive benefit to subjects, but ignore the real benefits that accrue
to researchers. Despite the fact that he or she stands to gain professional advancement and stature, research funding, outright
payments, fame, and prizes, the researcher's opinion and behaviors are assumed to be "objective" and are often cast as unalloyed
beneficence. Donna Haraway captures this when she writes:

> [Scientists] tell parables about objectivity and scientific
> method to students in the first years of their initiation. . . .
> [Their] gaze claims the power to see and not be seen, to rep-
> resent while escaping representation. This gaze signifies the
> unmarked positions of Man and White, one of the many nasty
> tones of the word "objectivity."

The scientific stance requires objective assessment of
potential benefits and risks, and if informed consent had been
required, the researchers would have to share with subjects the
fact that hypothermia is an often-fatal medical crisis and the
weak rationale for suggesting that hypothermia will improve
their chances of survival. Wariness would ensue, especially
if they learned that Tisherman would personally profit from
their ordeal.

Then there is also the ethical question of clinical equipoise, which requires a genuine uncertainty on the part of the

110   medical researcher and community whether the risks of pro-
       found hypothermia, with its 40 percent death rate (diminished
       further when subjects are also injured, as these men are), will
       be more beneficial than the standard of care that doesn't carry
       such risks.

       African Americans suffer disproportionately higher rates
       of disease, injury, and death caused by higher rates of poverty,
       toxic environments, stress (including the stress of racism),
       and reduced access to medical care, including reduced access
       to existing approved technologies like transplant and approved
       heart therapies. It is ethically noxious to exploit their phys-
       ical vulnerability due to a racially biased healthcare system
       by exposing them to the risk of a hazardous experiment while
       sparing others the dangers of this dubious trial. This violates
       the ethical precept of distributive justice because the risks and
       potential benefits are stratified by race—today. Tomorrow, the
       risks will face all Americans as nonconsensual research—for
       profit—becomes more normalized

       Baltimore was home to Henrietta Lacks, whose valuable
       cells were appropriated by researchers over the strident objec-
       tions of her husband. It is also home to the only documented
       burking (a murder in order to sell the body to anatomists) in
       the United States. Baltimore is also where public-health agen-
       cies stand accused of spreading "treated" human waste on the
       lawns of inner-city homes and of encouraging landlords of lead-
       tainted housing to rent to families with small children in order
       to test the effectiveness of low-cost lead abatement by mon-
       itoring lead levels in the children's blood. All this was done
       without informed consent.

How sadly fitting that this city, and our nation, should harbor such an egregious and racially dichotomous human-rights violation of a type that is burgeoning and encoded into law.

But in such studies victims of color are often, as a Maryland appellate court has pointed out, "the canaries in the coal mine," because the contemporary challenge to informed consent is one that threatens us all.

Pushing "Special K"

As he headed to a Kentucky veterans' national convention in late August 2019, President Donald Trump let fly the sort of off-the-cuff, data-free utterance that has launched a thousand facepalms.

"There's a product that's made right now that just came out by Johnson & Johnson," he enthused, "which has a tremendously positive—pretty short term, but nevertheless positive—effect." The commander in chief announced that he'd instructed the Department of Veterans Affairs to make a large purchase of Spravato, the brand name of the ketamine derivative called esketamine. He praised esketamine as a "stimulant" that would address the widespread epidemic of depression among veterans.

But ketamine and its variants, including esketamine, the "left-handed" form of the ketamine molecule, are the precise opposite of a stimulant. Ketamine is a potent *depressant*, used in both human and veterinary surgery as a general anesthetic. This powerful hallucinogen also induces dreamlike states, dissociation, hallucinations; sedation; confusion; loss of memory;

raised blood pressure; unconsciousness; dangerously slowed breathing; seizures; and a lingering disruption of attention, learning, and memory. Its long-term effects range from ravaged kidneys to the very depression that VA doctors are trying to banish.

Ketamine, a class III schedule drug, is so powerful and its side effects so dangerous that its medical uses have long been restricted to surgery under expert anesthesiologists' care in carefully monitored and controlled conditions.

Ketamine is also better known by its subterranean alter ego: "Special K," or simply "K," a powerfully addictive street drug. The National Institute on Drug Abuse warns that "there are no FDA-approved medications to treat addiction to ketamine or other dissociative drugs." Ketamine is even slipped to the unsuspecting as a notorious date-rape drug, thanks to the stupor, unconsciousness, and memory loss it induces.

Some researchers explain that in seeking answers for stubborn problems like veterans' high depression and suicide rate, they wish to expand the legitimate medical uses of some drugs beyond narrow applications like ketamine's strictly surgical role. However, when the FDA greenlighted expedited clinical trials to test esketamine against depression over several years, six people who had been administered the drug died, as opposed to no deaths among subjects who took placebos. In June, just a few months before Trump's directive, the Veterans Administration's medical advisory board was unimpressed enough to vote against including esketamine in the formulary list of drugs that its hospital system offers.

Emails procured by ProPublica revealed that at his Mar-a-Lago resort, three of Trump's friends were working with

114   Johnson & Johnson and the VA on veterans' depression and suicide as the company's drug was being developed. Trump subsequently touted Spravato's "incredible" effectiveness in a June 12
meeting with VA Secretary Robert Wilkie, and offered to help
the VA negotiate its purchase.

Despite the desultory trial results, the FDA did approve
Spravato, although only with the concomitant use of an oral
antidepressant medication and with a dire "black box" warning
about serious risks associated with the drug, and only for
treating severe depression. The doctors of the watchdog group
Public Citizen took issue with the approval, writing: "Disturbingly, the FDA appears to inappropriately discount the possibility that these suicides were linked to esketamine exposure."

The FDA's industry-friendly tendency to approve drugs
like esketamine, even when evidence suggests the possibility
of inordinate harm, is something critics have long decried,
including some experts who work within the FDA. As one FDA
medical evaluator wrote in response to a 1998 Public Citizen
survey, "My feeling after more than twenty years at FDA is that
unless drugs can be shown to kill patients outright then they
will be approved with revised labeling and box warning." The
Spravato labeling does indeed contain such a boxed warning
that cautions that patients are at risk for sedation and difficulty
with attention, judgment, and thinking (dissociation), abuse
and misuse, and suicidal thoughts and behaviors.

Another FDA scientist concurred, writing, "We are in the
midst now to approve everything but to describe drug weak-
nesses in the label." As one high-ranking official said, "Everything is approvable. We can use the labeling creatively to lower
the problems."

Why did the Trump administration go to the trouble of seeking FDA approval for esketamine when ketamine was already FDA-approved, its action is similar to esketamine, and it is in common use? Why not simply use ketamine?

Because ketamine is off-patent—and thus has lost its exclusivity for FDA-approved uses, resulting in plummeting profits. Esketamine, the new variant, sold as Spravato, is patented—and potentially lucrative, should a large-enough market be found. The vast military market would do nicely, and so would an expansion of its uses beyond surgery, into the practice of "treating" suicides and depression

Esketamine's use to address milder conditions such as depression or even for calming the agitated would also serve to expand the sedatives market and inflate its profits. This is what's called function creep, in which a contested technology or policy with a narrowly focused application expands into common use. (For example, forcible DNA collection from criminals was originally confined to one of the most heinous subsets of convicted violent offenders: child molesters. But by 2020, New York State had amassed 82,000 DNA profiles as it mandated DNA collection from anyone, even a child, who was questioned about a crime.)

Completing the right clinical trials successfully could allow ketamine to become more profitable, too. Finding a new use for ketamine entails having a new study in order to have it approved by the FDA. But before the research study can be conducted, its protocol—the detailed blueprint for conducting it—must be approved by the institutional review board (IRB), to ensure that it meets medical and ethical and legal requirements. The board consists of experts and at least one additional member who

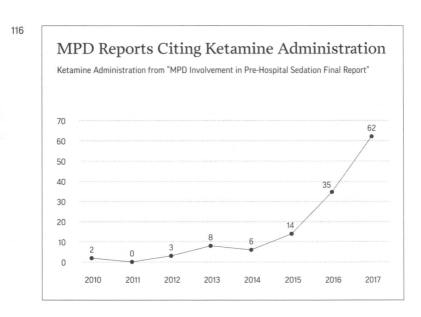

MPD Reports Citing Ketamine Administration

Ketamine Administration from "MPD Involvement in Pre-Hospital Sedation Final Report"

must be unaffiliated with the research organization or medical center. The IRB bears responsibility for protecting subjects' health, dignity, and welfare and for scrutinizing the study's scientific, logical, and risk-benefit analysis. The IRB must also ensure that the study adheres to federal laws and ethical strictures. The federal government is supposed to oversee IRBs, but this oversight rarely occurs, making IRBs only as effective and ethical as the members who constitute them. Some IRBs permit grievous abuses and scientific lapses. For example, IRBs have approved giving young New York City boys the cardiotoxic drug fenfluramine as part of a violence study and of deliberately exposing young children in Baltimore to lead—even going so far as to advise the researchers on how to skirt federal requirements, according to the Maryland appellate court ruling.

After gaining IRB approval, the trail can be carried out in an attempt to gain FDA approval. The FDA, an agency within the Department of Health and Human Services (HHS), regulates clinical tests of medications, biologicals, and medical devices, in concert with the Office for Human Research Protections (OHRP), which protects the rights and welfare of human subjects in federally funded medical experimentation.

If the FDA approves the new use of ketamine, it may be sold at higher prices. The city of Minneapolis is an epicenter for such an expansion. Its medical institutions, including Hennepin Medical Center, today conduct human experimentation that may dramatically expand ketamine's market, at the cost of unwitting research subjects' health and right to informed consent—indeed, to any type of consent.

On December 16, 2017, Brittany Buckley, wracked with sobs, downed drink after drink, and then called a friend, Ron, to confess that she felt depressed and paralyzed by grief. It was nine days before Christmas, and Minneapolis was blanketed in photogenic snow. It was also the two-year anniversary of Brittany's father's death. Brittany couldn't stop thinking that her family could never reunite.

After calling Ron, Brittany laid silent and unmoving on her sofa. When Ron called to check on her, she didn't answer, and as he headed to her apartment, he called 911, explaining that Brittany was despondent over her father's death. Soon, he met officers John Bennett and James Lynch at her apartment. Using Ron's key, they entered.

After rousing Brittany and speaking with her briefly, the police called an ambulance. Three paramedics responded and

quickly decided that she should go to the hospital. Brittany dis-
agreed, and asked the paramedics to leave.

According to a complaint her lawyers filed, paramedic
Anthony D'Agostino "stated that she was on a medical trans-
portation hold and would have to come with them." Brittany
reiterated her refusal to go to the hospital, and in response,
paramedics and the police pulled her to her feet, "handcuffed
her behind her back, and carried her out of the building and into
the ambulance. Ms. Buckley never attempted to kick, strike, or
bite anyone as she was being carried out to the ambulance."

The complaint stated that as Brittany was rolled onto her
back, both arms cuffed to the gurney and strapped down by
shoulder harness and hip, thigh, and ankle straps, she cried and
continually stated that she did not want to go to the hospital,
but never physically resisted the police, ambulance personnel,
or the restraints.

The ambulance attendants' report paints a different picture:
"Patient attempted kicking, biting, and headbutting responders
while she was being removed from her house and taken to the
ambulance," it reads. "It was elect[ed to] enroll her into the
ketamine trials." However, camera recordings from cameras
mounted on the bodies of officers Bennett and Lynch contra-
dict the report, and so does the ambulance-run record created
by paramedics D'Agostino, Katherine A. Kaufmann, and Jonathan R. Thomalia. These show that Brittany engaged in verbal
outbursts but was not physically aggressive or combative.

Nevertheless, having described her behavior as qualifying
on the study's scale that measured agitation, the paramedics
enrolled her in a ketamine trial, which meant that they injected
her with a drug-filled syringe. They did not ask her permission,

did not tell her that she was now enrolled in a medical experiment, nor did they identify the ketamine that they were forcing
on her.

Moreover, an account by Andy Mannix, who writes for the
Minneapolis Star Tribune, denies that Brittany met the study
criteria:

> On a scale the hospital uses to judge a person's agitation
> levels, a "plus-four" means "severely agitated." Buckley was a
> "plus-two," according to her medical records, which she shared
> with the *Star Tribune*. Paramedics noted that she appeared
> "agitated" and "anxious" but was attentive and smiling.

As Brittany watched them prepare the injection, she
objected verbally to it.

Brittany was forcibly injected as a subject in "Ketamine
versus Midazolam for Prehospital Agitation," a study into ketamine's possible use to quell agitation when injected by paramedics in ambulances. According to the complaint, "This was
the second of two Hennepin County studies attempting to vali-
date the use of ketamine by ambulance crews to sedate patients
whom paramedics deemed agitated. In this study, agitation
was defined as 'a state of extreme emotional disturbance where
patients become physically aggressive or violent, endangering
themselves or those caring for them.'"

In an earlier study, "A Prospective Study of Ketamine
versus Haloperidol for Severe Prehospital Agitation," paramedics assessed patients against an Altered Mental Status
Scale (AMSS), an internal Hennepin Healthcare Systems, Inc.,
measurement tool based on a combination of other scales.

120   These purport to measure alertness, intoxication, sedation, or agitation.

The study's publicity conflates research with treatment when it indicates that "Hennepin EMS has been using ketamine as the standard of care for patients safely since 2008." But ketamine is not the standard of care for such agitation, neither was Brittany a patient. What she underwent was not treatment. Although the ketamine injection was described as an attempt to help Brittany by controlling her agitation and resistant behavior, ketamine is not approved for this use. Its use here was not therapy, but research, and Brittany was not a patient but a research subject.

The distinction is not empty semantics, because patients enjoy rights and a status that research subjects do not. The purpose of medical treatment is to enhance an individual patient's health and welfare. The patient's well-being is the focus of, and the very reason for, treatment.

But in medical research, the focus is the successful conduct of the research and the gleaning, aggregation, and analysis of information from it. An individual subject is primarily a means to an end. The researcher may hope that the experimental modality will improve the individual subject's health, but the real beneficiary is other patients—including future patients who may benefit from research revelations.

Moreover, Brittany had been forced into this research without notification, without her permission, and despite the objections that everyone agrees she repeatedly voiced. How could this be? Doesn't U.S. law protect people from being coerced into medical research without their consent?

Since 1996, being forced to participate in medical research has been permitted under the Federal Code of Regulations statute CFR 21 50.23-4, provided certain conditions are met. One of those conditions is that the prospective subject must be a trauma victim, based upon the assumption that such subjects are unconscious and incapable of giving (or withholding) consent.

Brittany, however, was indeed conscious and objected, many times, so she could not be forced into research under this law.

But the fact that she was conscious and objected did not preclude her forcible participation because researchers used yet another end run around consent, also enacted in 1996. This waiver of consent is provided by a different section of the Code of Federal Regulations: 45 CFR 46.116, which gives "IRBs authority to alter or waive the required consent in certain circumstances, typically when researchers claim the research does not involve human subjects research or when they claim it entails only 'minimal risk.'"

When her ambulance reached the Hennepin County Medical Center, Brittany was diagnosed with acute hypoxia (low oxygen) and respiratory failure, which is often caused by the ketamine injection. To ensure that she could breathe, she had to be intubated until the following day, a procedure that carries risks of life-threatening complications: More than one in four intubated people suffer severe hypoxaemia, an abnormally low concentration of oxygen in the blood. One in twenty goes into cardiac arrest.

Brittany woke up the next day with a document that had been left for her to sign. At the top of the paper was "Consent for Clinical Investigation Conducted with Patient's Notification

122 of Enrollment." It belatedly asked her consent to enroll in the experiment, but assured her that she could refuse participation, which meant that the data collected from her would not be used. Of course, the definition of "consent" precludes obtaining it *after* one has been used in a research study. "They tell people afterward that they can opt out of the study if they wish and their data will not be used," Carl Elliott told me by telephone. "The problem is, there is no real opting out." Elliott is a professor in the Center for Bioethics and the Departments of Pediatrics and Philosophy at the University of Minnesota. He added, "Subjects' objection is not to their data being used. Their objection is to waking up in the hospital on a ventilator after being injected with ketamine."

In September 2019, a federal judge dismissed Brittany's lawsuit. But many more lawsuits are pending in four separate Minnesota ketamine experiments involving dozens of people sedated by paramedics, many at the urging of police.

One such complaint has been brought by Katie Hosley on behalf of her and her son Thomas "Trey" Hosley.

In late October 2017, seventeen-year-old Trey and a few friends bought some LSD and went to his home to take it. Something went wrong.

"It was about midnight and I remember [Trey's friend] waking me and saying, 'Something's wrong with Trey; he's having a seizure, I think,'" Katie told me. "So I called the paramedics. I didn't call the police. But when the first responders arrived, they were accompanied by police, and the police were very belligerent. And they're the ones who scared him the most, I think."

"When I woke up, there were four cops in the room," Trey told me. "Then I blacked out; I'm told I had a seizure. When I came to, three cops were on top of me. My mother rushed forward to stop them, and a woman punched my mom. I don't really know why."

"She hit me in my chest and pushed me backward," said Katie. "She said that I was high or something. And just so you know, I have never done a drug in my life. And even if I was, that's really not her business. But I wasn't."

"I blacked out as soon as I saw that," said Trey. "When I was blacked out is when they hit me with the ketamine."

"We have all of these officers who kill innocent people and whatever. And I'm terrified and I'm thinking, 'Are they going to do the same type of thing to my son?'" Katie told me. "My son, who is the most gentle giant you could ever meet—but he's also African American." Katie is not.

Katie said she asked the EMTs to take Trey to nearby Abbott Northwestern Hospital, where all of their health records are kept. They refused, saying, "No, we're taking him to HCMC [Hennepin County Medical Center]." When she asked why, "Finally one first responder kind of pulled me aside and said, 'He's being enrolled in a ketamine study. We're taking him to HCMC,'" she said. "But I didn't understand it at the time, because I had never even heard of it"

The next day, Trey remembers waking up in the HCMC, a Level-I trauma center. There are five levels of U.S. trauma care, ranked according to the types of resources they boast and the number of patients they accommodate annually. According to the American Trauma Society, the nation's Level-I centers

124   can care "for every aspect of injury from prevention through rehabilitation."

"They told me if I could eat something and drink some water, I could leave earlier," Trey said. "I didn't want to stay there for long, so I ate whatever they gave me and drank a cup of water, and I got to leave."

No one told him he'd been injected with ketamine. "I kind of just figured I had overdosed. They kept recommending that I go to drug treatment. They gave me a piece of paper, but they didn't really mention too much what it was for." Once Trey returned home, he said he didn't feel the same. "My body hurt real bad. I've never had a pain like that throughout my body. For a week straight it just kept going on. I couldn't feel my thumb; I couldn't feel that for a good seven months because they pinched my nerve really tightly. I started taking meth, and am just now getting over a year-long meth addiction."

Sixty-four doctors, bioethicists, and academics were alarmed enough by these and other misrepresentations to join medical watchdog group Public Citizen in signing a letter to the FDA and the Office for Human Research Protections (OHRP) that urged an investigation into the conduct of the clinical trials.

"I think I make poorer decisions now than I did before," Trey said. "It's not right what they did to me without asking."

Erasing Consent

What precisely is informed consent? Most of us have a notion, however vague, that in twenty-first-century America, patients can't be coerced into medical research without their permission, and that this permission must be not only voluntary but also informed by a useful knowledge of what the research entails. Many people, and even some healthcare workers, consider informed consent a piece of paper, a document signed by the subject to indicate her understanding of the study's purpose, requirements, and other pertinent details, including known risks.

But informed consent is much more than a piece of paper. Informed consent helps to enforce ethical principles of autonomy, beneficence, and justice, and the signed form is only one piece of evidence buttressing a researcher's claim that she has explained everything a subject reasonably needs to know in order to make the best decision about whether he wants to participate. The researcher should impart information guided by

126   the question: What would the average patient need to know to be an informed participant in the decision? She also should bear in mind the question: What would a typical physician say about this research study?

The subject must be provided information about the study's purpose, requirements, design, known risks, possible discomfort, and putative benefits. Subjects must be informed of all their options in addition to participating in the study, including the option to take an approved, tested treatment, to pursue nonpharmaceutical treatment instead, or to pursue no treatment at all. The exchange is confidential except that FDA staff may read it. The protocol, or blueprint for the medical research, must lay out and explain whether compensation or treatment will be provided for adverse events, and that the subject can leave the study at any time, whether she has been paid or not. Contact information must be provided for a staff person to consult, in case further questions arise.

Informed consent also means warning the subject about possible lifestyle effects. Will he be fatigued? Feel discomfort? Be unable to sleep, or to drive? Informed consent is continuous, not static, so any developments or discoveries that emerge throughout the study, such as adverse effects that might impinge upon a subject's decision to continue in the study, must be shared with the subjects. The responsibility to communicate this information persists throughout the study so that subjects must be warned about, for example, any dangerous effects that emerge during the study.

As mentioned earlier, informed consent can manifest quite differently when a patient is considering treatment than when a subject is considering enrolling in research.

In general, informed consent is required for treatment, for dissemination of patient information, for discussion of HIPAA laws, specific procedures, surgery, blood transfusions, and anesthesia. In a situation where a patient faces serious illness or death but is unable to communicate his wishes, a doctor can justify dispensing with informed consent because it is reasonable to infer or assume that the patient would want to be treated. It is reasonable to assume that a sick or injured man who walks into an emergency room but faints before he can ask for help has done so because he wishes to be treated. It is reasonable to assume that a woman who collapses on the street would want a nearby physician to treat her—or even a trained layperson to administer CPR. This *presumed consent* is why laws exist to protect healthcare workers, and sometimes bystanders, who attempt to aid the ill in emergencies.

However, we cannot make the same logical assumption that the fainting woman would welcome the attentions of a bystander who sprinkles herbs or snake oil on her to see if that would help her recover, or that she would want a nearby physician to inject artificial blood into her veins or to test on her an experimental do-it-yourself resuscitation device he has constructed out of LEGOs.

The latter scenarios would present a research situation, not approved treatment. The distinction between treatment and research is an important one. Approved treatments are relatively effective and safe, with risks that have been adjudged acceptable given the demonstrated proven benefits of treatment. By contrast, research modalities—herbs, snake oil, artificial blood, or homemade resuscitation devices—have not been proven safe or beneficial.

Moreover, there is the often-overlooked distinction between patients and research subjects. The goal of treatment
for a patient is to maximize that specific patient's health and
well-being. Drug selection, precise dosage, and adjustments in
treatment are made with the prime goal of achieving the best
outcome for the individual patient. The focus of research is not
the best outcome for an individual subject, but rather the successful completion of the experiment. Although a researcher
may *hope* for an optimal outcome for each individual subject,
drug selection and dosage is typically determined by computer
randomization with the successful study, not subject health.
Researchers will seek to limit harms by, for example, truncating
a study in which subjects are suffering unacceptable levels of
harm or deaths. But research subjects are not patients, a term
that denotes a therapeutic relationship that does not exist
between a subject and a study's researchers.

After the Second World War, the Nuremburg Code was
imposed to ban research without voluntary consent. Informed
consent was enshrined into U.S. law in 1947 to ensure that
research would never be imposed on Americans without their
knowledge or consent. Although the nonconsensual experimental abuse continued, especially with groups such as
African Americans. It was often done secretly, as when scientists injected subjects with toxic plutonium. At other times,
researchers lied about having procured informed consent, as
when Eugene Saenger subjected cancer sufferers to total body
irradiation in Cincinnati without their knowledge and with fatal
results, even though their cancers were known to resist radiation. Or they lied about the experimental nature of the medical

attention, falsely claiming or implying experimental medications and techniques were approved therapy.

The conflicts of interest rife in the medical industry extend to some ethicists, who one might expect to decry the divided loyalties of institutions, medical centers, and pharmaceutical companies. Many ethicists receive checks and academic appointments from, and sit on the boards of, the research institutions that they ostensibly monitor, so their interests are closely aligned with the institutions they shy away from condemning.

Procuring informed consent makes the lengthy and expensive process of human medical research even more time-consuming, and the FDA permits only a few years to complete the clinical trial process. Moreover, it can be hard to convince subjects who meet trial criteria to join trials. This is not only true of marginalized groups; mainstream Americans harbor a great deal of distrust as well. And the nature of many trials can be discouraging: Many trials are unsavory, dangerous, or simply sound distasteful.

But by 1995, U.S. medical research had found a way around informed consent: waivers. Researchers who wanted to avoid the trouble and expense of individual informed consent for medical research would ask the federal government to waive the requirement to elicit consent from large groups of potential subjects such as soldiers, who were used to test experimental anthrax and pyridostigmine injections and artificial blood. In time, some researchers also found this piecemeal process of securing waivers for individual studies burdensome. They clamored for a yet easier way of eluding consent.

As mentioned in Chapter Three, in 1996 addenda to the Code of Federal Regulations achieved two legal means of avoiding consent. One, for research under 45 CFR. 46.116 (d), provides a waiver of consent on the basis that the study provides "no more than minimal risk to the subjects" as when agitated Minnesota patients are injected with ketamine by EMTS in ambulances. This is also invoked when researchers claim that the study does not entail human subjects research at all, but, for example, was merely documentation or recordkeeping.

The other amendment, 21 CFR 50.23-24, is applied to experiments that are acknowledged as human subjects research, like infusing trauma victims with concentrated saline of artificial blood or testing patented valves for use in cardiopulmonary respiration (CPR). However, informed consent (actually, consent of any type) is dispensed with because the subject is a trauma victim who is gravely injured, presumed unconscious, and therefore unable to give consent.

For-Profit IRBs Cash In

Some insist that nonconsensual research is safe because institutional research boards sufficiently protect U.S. research participants. However, IRBs have their limitations.

"Expedited review" by IRBs permits evaluation by a few or sometimes only a single member. And the law requires only a single member who is unaffiliated with the institution. This provides insufficient representation of the people who will comprise the subject pool and bear the risks of research.

Worse, many medical and policy experts concerned with clinical trial safety express alarm by the trend away from evaluation by university-based IRBs and toward assessment by for-profit IRBs—also referred to as *contract research organizations* (CROs). The U.S. Government Accounting Office also expressed alarm.

CRO advertisements to researchers and medical institutions focus on the delivery of quick, positive results: Some seemed to virtually promise fast approvals. But are they performing the role of an IRB? That is, are they engaged in due diligence, and adequately protecting research subjects by investigating the safety, risk-benefit analysis, and conformity to ethical standards and applicable laws? One CRO, Coast Independent Review Board of Colorado Springs, reviewed 356 research proposals within five years and rejected only one. The high acceptance rate proved profitable: Its revenue doubled to $9.3 million within that period. According to the *Wall Street Journal,* Coast directly or indirectly reviewed studies for the majority of the world's largest pharmaceutical companies, medical-device makers, and biotechnology companies.

Rules, laws, and federal experts exist to guide IRBs, but the oversight dictated by law is rarely performed, so that an IRB is as effective and ethical as its members. And conflict of interest is built into the system, because a CRO's profits are directly dependent upon satisfying the makers of the product it tests.

In 2009, the House Subcommittee on Investigations and Oversight decided to conduct a sting. It devised a fictitious proposal by Device Med-Systems to pump at least a liter of a gelatinous substance it called Adhesiabloc directly into the abdomens of women patients undergoing surgery, ostensibly to discourage the formation of surgical adhesions that can cause post-surgery complications or complicate later surgeries. The Adhesiabloc substance was not precisely defined, making it impossible to evaluate its safety. The principal investigator, who is ultimately responsible for the study design and conduct, was also fictitious: Dr. Jonathan Q. Kruger, a Virginia physician with a four-page *curriculum vitae* and a medical license that had expired eighteen years earlier (although a number of other duly credentialed physicians by that name practice in the U.S.). The address for the institution where the clinical trials were to take place was a post-office box in a strip mall in Clifton, Virginia.

In addition to the nonexistent company, the imaginary, undefined product, and the uncredentialed doctor, the GAO sprinkled ample clues throughout the proposal. "Phake Medical Devices'" given address was another post-office box, in Chetesville, Arizona; Staffers April Phuls, Timothy Witless, and Alan Ruse all made appearances.

But was anyone paying attention? Fortunately, yes. Two CROs to whom the GAO submitted the phony proposal—Argus Independent Review Board, of Tucson, and Fox Commercial Institutional Review Board, of Springfield, Illinois—rejected it outright, dismissing the trial as "awful" and "a piece of junk."

However, Coast approved it. Its review panel unanimously approved the fake protocol that entailed pouring a full liter of the fictitious product into a woman's stomach after surgery. According to the minutes of the board meeting at which the Adhesiabloc protocol was approved, all board members thought the product was "probably very safe."

But Coast had no empirical basis for this claim. Not only had it failed to discover that the products and researchers described by the protocol were nonexistent, it failed to discern or even to discuss the study's very significant risk to subjects. It did not know the composition of Adhesiabloc, and did not sufficiently consider the risk of introducing a large quantity of any substance into the abdomen of surgical patients. Higher-risk studies should trigger greater-than-usual scrutiny and an analysis of whether they are justified in the light of potential benefits. If approved, such protocols must include disclosure of known side effects, and mechanisms for monitoring and the reporting of adverse events—none of which were required by Coast.

Coast's approval spurred an invitation to Coast CEO Daniel Dueber from the U.S. House Committee on Energy and Commerce Subcommittee on Oversight in March 2009 to explain his company's decision. Coast then realized there was a problem with the proposal, belatedly researched it, and discovered the deception.

Dueber pushed back by questioning the government sting's legality and ethics and casting his company as victims of government deceit. "I cannot believe that my government did this to me and my company," said Dueber. "It is unconscionable."

After the GOA probe and hearings, an unimpressed FDA issued a warning letter to Coast on April 14. A number of Coast's "key customers" then defected, and after initially announcing plans to reorganize, Coast declared bankruptcy and decided to close. It subsequently passed three hundred clinical trials on to other IRBs and CROs to evaluate—hopefully using much more diligence than had Coast.

The Coast sting illustrates not only the continuing dangers of for-profit CROs but also the conflicts of interest inherent in traditional IRBs, whose existence and funding depends upon the institutions whose proposals they evaluate.

134   **"It's Very Rare"**

Why are many medical ethicists, who had held informed consent as sacred for at least half a century, unconcerned about contemporary human medical research that dispenses with it altogether?

In 2006, while a nonconsensual clinical trial of the artificial blood substitute PolyHeme study was still underway, my search for answers led me to the office of Daniel K. Nelson, PhD, Director of the EPA's Human Research Protocol and University of North Carolina-Chapel Hill Center for Bioethics. At the time we met, Nelson had supervised at least seven IRBs that had judged at least four thousand research studies.

Nelson helped federal drafters to evaluate, refine, and eventually to accept the 21 CFR 50.24 exception that allows medical researchers to bypass informed consent. Was there no way, I asked, to test untried modalities other than to use the injured without their knowledge?

"It's an emergency where people are likely to be unconscious and unable to give consent," he observed evenly. "What would you suggest?"

I suggested that dispensing with consent reflected a curious lack of imagination, because other medical trauma policies have preferred opt-in schemes that notified potential participants of the details of a medical procedure, then allowed medical personnel to secure true consent in emergency scenarios.

For example, there's the "opt-in" procedure that we use to procure organs for transplant. First, we saturate an area with informational messages such as posters and public-service announcements announcing the critical need for donated organs, and then we provide the means for opting in. These include the

familiar signing of a driver's license or an organ-donor card. In
testing artificial blood, for example, we could allow the same
signing of one's license or offer PolyHeme-acceptance cards for
voluntary signature, just as we sign organ-donor cards today. This
would provide experimental access to the informed and willing
and would avoid robbing people of their autonomy and consent.

"First of all, organ donation isn't research," Nelson counters,
"and the PolyHeme study takes place in an emergency situation
where the person is unconscious."

But organ harvesting, like infusing PolyHeme, also takes
place in emergency situations where persons are dead, brain-
dead, unconscious under general anesthesia, or otherwise
unable to give consent. Organ donation is not research, but
that doesn't matter, I insist, because this manner of procuring
organs offers a model of eliciting consent in emergency situations, a model that works.

This opt-in approach could be adapted to many scenarios.
If we were testing ways to treat people suffering the sort of
traumas that result from motor vehicle accidents, we could
identify, educate, and ask advance permission of people who are
most likely to suffer such injuries—for example, motorcyclists
or drivers of all-terrain vehicles. If we wished to test stroke
remedies, we could identify at-risk people with hypertension,
obesity, genetic predispositions, or other elevated risks and do
the same. A touch ghoulish, perhaps, but far less so than forcing
them into experiments without their permission.

Nelson's brow wrinkled, then he paused. "I'll think about
that one," he said, and smiled.

"You know," he offered genially, while leaning forward
slightly, "in 1996, when the rules changed, we discussed the

exception proposal at length; we agonized over it, over the language and protections. When we finalized the legislation, we braced ourselves for an onslaught of proposals to use the exception, but they never came. It's very rarely used. In ten years the use of exceptions has been approved approximately ten times by the emergency medicine folks. Studies utilizing the waiver have never been numerous, and the few that transpired get a lot of attention."

Nelson is not the first to offer, not ethical justifications, but an invocation of how rare the exceptionalism is.

Except that, these legal exceptions had been used not ten, but a minimum of fifteen times at the time we spoke, although no exact count exists. They did not always go smoothly, according to published reports in the medical literature.

As North Carolina lawyer Nancy King observed in 2007, "The emergency-consent exception is supposed to carve out a very narrow window. What's been happening is that narrow window seems to be expanding."

Now, the window has been thrown wide open. An experimental anthrax vaccine and drugs were forced on approximately 900,000 military troops. The subjects of at least fifteen EFICs enrolling 45,000 people over the past two decades included the 720 trauma subjects in the PolyHeme study. Its principal investigator, Myron Weisfeldt, told me the Research Outcomes Consortium (ROC), an ambitious research partnership, is on track toward its goal of enrolling 22,000 unwitting subjects in Seattle, Iowa, Portland, San Diego, Dallas, Birmingham, Pittsburgh, Milwaukee, Toronto, Ottawa, and British Columbia.

No one can now call legal research without consent "rare."

The drafters may have *intended* consent-free trials to be rare, but their burgeoning should surprise no one: It is a predictable example of function creep.

I ask Nelson to describe some of the prior 50.23 studies he alluded to, but he can remember only one, he says.

"There's the AED [automated external defibrillator], which was approved in such a study. Before then, defibrillators were only used by trained personnel in emergency settings—such as hospitals and ambulances. We wondered, 'What if they were in public areas and directions allowed laypersons to use them: Would this save lives?' But you could not procure informed consent, because you cannot predict when someone will suffer cardiac arrest."

Sudden cardiac arrest, occurring when the coordinated electrical signals that generate an orderly, regular heartbeat become deranged, results in ventricular fibrillation. The heart falls into arrhythmia, then suddenly stops. This is caused by electrical malfunction, and applying electric shock to the heart via a defibrillator can restore a healthy rhythm. Of the 350,000 people felled by cardiac arrest outside hospitals each year, only 5 percent are saved, but this number rises to 50 percent or more in those who are immediately shocked.

"We conducted research and found that, indeed, yes, AEDs save lives," recalls Nelson. "Now there are defibrillators in airports, planes, and malls."

Public Misunderstanding

It is a persuasive example. Results of the study published in the *New England Journal of Medicine* in 2004 found that, of the 235

138   heart-attack victims treated, 30 who received both defibrilla-
       tion and CPR survived, but only 15 survived after receiving CPR
       alone. The experiment saved lives and seemed to have no down-
       side, making the automatic external defibrillator the poster child
       for informed consent exceptionalism. It remains an oft-touted
       example of when research with the unwitting may be beneficial.

       The responses resembled those from a larger survey of
       public attitudes, conducted during the defibrillation trial.
       Terri A. Schmidt, professor of emergency medicine at Oregon
       Health and Science University, and Michelle Biros of the Uni-
       versity of Minnesota interviewed 530 people who were vis-
       iting or receiving treatment at two emergency rooms during
       the time the defibrillation study was enrolling patients in
       these cities. Responses suggested that members of the public
       might have become aware of the study through mandatory
       public-notification efforts that included newspaper advertise-
       ments and community meetings.

       Ninety percent of respondents thought informed consent
       should be mandatory. But when the survey asked specifically
       about the defibrillation trial, 70 percent said they had no objec-
       tion to that trial, even without being asked for consent.

       This apparent contradiction is neither inconsistent nor
       surprising, because the much-lauded AED study is not a typical
       example of nonconsensual research.

       Defibrillation could hardly differ more from experiments
       like those with the experimental anthrax vaccine forced on sol-
       diers or the dangerous and unapproved blood substitute Poly-
       Heme. Defibrillation is a proven therapeutic treatment with a
       good track record of safety and effectiveness, which people will
       accept in emergencies, rather than an experimental agent like

PolyHeme with a fatality-littered history, of which people are understandably more wary. Defibrillation, unlike anthrax shots or PolyHeme, is the standard of care.

In fact, one could argue that the AED study tested, not defibrillators, but the ability of laypersons to use them.

Moreover, despite the rosy depiction of putative benefits, not every such study of drugs and devices has a happy ending. We could not expect them to because they are research, not treatment: By definition, the benefits are not guaranteed and their outcomes are unpredictable. In fact, ethical principles dictate that if we knew one approach to be superior to the other, it would be wrong to run the test and subject some to what was known to be the inferior remedy. This is the concept of *equipoise*: The researcher must inhabit a genuine uncertainty about the superiority and tested modalities.

Some experimental devices harmed rather than helped, like an unnamed heart-assist device that was tested without consent and left disappointment and death in its wake. In 2006, the *Journal of American Medical Association* published the disastrous outcome of a nonconsensual experiment testing the device, which delivered chest compressions, in five cities. Emergency responders gave CPR to 1,071 research subjects whose hearts had stopped beating, either with or without the device. Ten percent of patients they gave regular CPR to, the standard of care, survived, but fewer than 6 percent of the patients who received CPR administered using the device lived. Use of the device cost twenty people their lives, but unfortunately the device remained in use.

Although Nelson didn't remember any other nonconsensual studies, my brief search revealed that the very first study to utilize the 50.23 loophole was a trial of HemeAssist (diaspirin cross-linked hemoglobin), which, like PolyHeme, was a blood substitute. It was manufactured by Baxter Corporation and heavily bankrolled by the military. Like PolyHeme, HemeAssist was given to unwitting trauma victims, but the study had to be stopped when these subjects died and suffered heart attacks in proportions far greater than those not given it. The 2008 JAMA meta-analysis mentioned earlier in this book showed that eight tested blood substitutes shared similar mechanisms and resulted in similar records of heart attacks and death in clinical trials.

When I asked about the ethical acceptability of involuntary testing of substances that proved more hazardous than the standard of care, Nelson responded, "The [50.23] law has added protections built in to offset the lack of individual consent."

"Such as substituting community consultation for informed consent?" I asked.

"I think that's reasonable, to impart information."

Except that "community consultation" gives no opportunity to change the study and it rarely seems successful in alerting targeted communities. By far the most fraught of the conditions imposed upon the nonconsensual PolyHeme study, the affected "community" was to be informed of the study's details and afforded the opportunity to offer feedback. This was supposed to compensate for informed consent, and in fact it was originally called, in an access of semantic duplicity, "community consent." Proponents did well to eventually remove "consent" from its name, because no consent exists. The research design and rationale and design is presented as a fait accompli using PowerPoint slides. There is no opportunity for attendees to suggest changes to the studies' conduct.

Researchers have replaced informed consent with other deceptive models shrouded in jargon meant to confer the illusion of consent in order to "recruit" large numbers of involuntary subjects and to conduct research. "Presumed consent," "deferred consent," and "proxy consent" describe popular research scenarios that are united by the subjects' inability to exercise consent—or refusal.

Community consultation is also a misnomer because only a tiny percentage of potential subjects, not a community, are informed, not "consulted." Moreover, the "community consultation" meetings are conducted in locations where few of the targeted people tend to go. Such meetings have been sparsely attended and so failed to notify affected communities of the study. Even the term "community" gives pause because the "community" does not identify itself as such: It is a geographic entity defined by the group that wants to use it to conduct research.

Glenn McGee, PhD, founder of the *American Journal of Bioethics*, was in 2006 director of the Alden March Bioethics Institute Albany (New York) Medical College where an arm of the PolyHeme artificial blood experiment was conducted, he wrote, "My own group's study at Albany Med—a phone study of more than ten thousand residents of that metro area—found that essentially no one knew anything about the trial or the substance, and another study found that those who were presented with the possibility that they might get the substance were quite adamant that they would not want to be involuntarily

142   enrolled—if at all." Concerns over such violations led several institutions, such as those in Boston and Albany, to drop out of the study.

News reports in several study cities, including San Antonio, televised what happened when a reporter posted at a busy downtown intersection at lunchtime asked each passerby, "Have you heard of the PolyHeme study?" Not one person had.

And Ross McKinney Jr., vice dean for research at Duke University School of Medicine, estimated that community consultations around Duke "reached about 450 people," which he acknowledged was only a "tiny fraction" of Durham County's eight million residents.

Before taking my leave of Nelson, I shared with him my concerns about the increased vulnerability of people in inner-city areas who recieve inferior-quality healthcare. The heart attacks, gunshot wounds, violent traumas that are addressed in emergency rooms and ambulances are not the sort of problems and milieux that foster a doctor-patient relationship, but these people are used without their knowledge to test risky blood substitutes.

"Do not these types of [traumatic] injuries make these the very people most likely to benefit?" asked Nelson.

"No," I responded, "because these urbanites live near hospitals where blood is available, so that even should PolyHeme work well and safely, it offers them no benefit over saline. This research is intended to benefit those who live a considerable distance from care—rural trauma victims and those on battlefields."

Nelson didn't demur, and after thanking him, I left.

Reclaiming
Choice

The events described in this volume display a discouraging erosion of consent to medical research, yet there's not space enough to address every troubling aspect of what we have lost as the sacred right to say *yes* or *no* to medical research slips through our blind fingers.

The ambulance, for example, is being surreptitiously transformed from a chariot of universal mercy to an agent of medical compulsion for those who live in the wrong areas of targeted cities. Racial bias and abuse, at home and abroad, has never been expunged from medical research and encouraged researcher habits of secrecy, appropriation, and deception that grease the wheels of coercion not only for marginalized groups, but for all of us. I've discussed the special vulnerability of prisoners to conscription into research, but this defenselessness extends to many others in the wide swaths of the American carceral state, such as juvenile-justice institutions, mental-care facilities, and even nursing homes.

But although this book doesn't encompass every aspect of eroding consent, what it does describe suggests answers. For example, even if a compelling argument were ever made for non-consensual medical research, our recent history illustrates our inability to carry it out properly. An utter lack of transparency, duplicity, outright lies, distorting conflicts of interest, ethical and legal lapses, and sometimes fraudulence and a shocking disregard for human health, as in the cases of the Coast IRB and the experimental anthrax vaccines, reveal our inadequacy.

Philosophical arguments aside, we're simply not ready to dispense with consent, and perhaps we never will be.

But consent has been whittled away not by successful ethical argument or by persuasion, but because the U.S. medical research system maintains subjects in a voiceless and uninformed state. The much-ballyhooed "comment periods" on pending legislation are poorly publicized, far too short, and inadequate in scope. Members of the general public rarely hear of them or understand how to weigh in. How many people knew of the *two* major changes to federal law that were passed in 1996 after "comment periods" supposedly opened them to popular criticism? This discussion transpired only among medical professionals

Even the conditions imposed as feeble substitutes for the protection of informed consent have been breached by a flawed system whose desultory oversight permits too many lapses. So that in suspending informed consent, we have introduced a new set of procedural failures.

For example, the condition that the nonconsenting subject must be a trauma victim assumes unconsciousness and the inability to consent—without providing any mechanism for ascertaining that this is the case. Nor is any procedure established to determine whether a family member or legally authorized representative could provide consent. Some have argued this doesn't matter because more than mere consciousness is required for the potential subject to understand the complexities of informed consent. But the regulations do not state this; moreover, an inability to understand nuanced understanding would preclude informed consent, but would not preclude giving—or withholding—simple consent.

What's more, no consideration seems to have been given to the normal alternative—that once deemed incapable of consent, the patient should be considered ineligible for research and simply treated with the best known care, as if there were no research study to worry about. Because early pre-enactment discussions of this policy took place only among the researchers who would benefit from the research, and not among the potential subjects who would bear the risks, we cannot know whether potential subjects would prefer in such cases to be treated like patients, with treatment tailored to maximizing their individual health, or like research subjects, with medical acts rigidly focused on completing the study to gain information that furthers scientific knowledge.

Another ignored legal condition is that, to protect the subject, experimental treatment must stop when the approved therapeutic care becomes available and be replaced by approved care that is known to work. The PolyHeme study flouted this requirement to pursue the aims of the study. Researchers continued forcing experimental liquid on subjects for twelve hours after they reached the hospital, where blood was available. They

146   did this despite the excess deaths that plagued the earlier ANH hospital study of PolyHeme.

The requirement to notify people living in areas where they could become forced into medical experiments is too vague in that it doesn't stipulate whether the input will be used to change the study. In consequence, the study design has been presented to the relatively few residents who participated as a fait accompli. Perhaps more egregious, this study was conducted and allowed to proceed, even though it violated the North Carolina Patient Bill of Rights that guarantees informed consent in medical research.

Consent must be restored to American medical research. Recognize the right of every person to say *yes* or *no* as an absolute value and cease designating groups such as soldiers, unconscious emergency room patients, and Third World experimental subjects as appropriate subjects without their consent. When physicians are faced with a patient who is unable to consent to research and whose condition requires treatment before a family member or other proxy can be consulted, I propose that the patient be treated as if the physician had no research protocol to worry about. Don't enroll that patient in a study. Instead, use the best known treatment for that particular individual.

I submit that the two 1996 addenda to the Code of Federal Regulations that transformed medical research by tabling informed consent were improperly adopted without popular input and they should be revoked. Consent should not be marginalized on a national basis without a transparent national discussion followed by a referendum to elicit a clear and compelling mandate from the American public—from whom the subject pool is drawn—in order to go forward.

Who Watches These Watchers?

Given the revelations in this book, it will surprise no one that I favor this restoration of consent, but still more is needed to protect Americans against research conscription.

The IRBs that are supposed to evaluate human medical research have greenlighted too many unacceptable studies, from Coast's rubber-stamping of a risk-laden fictitious study to the approval of the Baltimore KKI lead study that exposed some children to hazardous lead, prompting a Maryland appellate court to chide the IRB for helping researchers to elude federal regulations.

Reforming IRBs

Among the issues that IRBs must better address are:

Conflicts of Interest

Financial conflicts of interest are rife in medical research. Some are sanctioned by law and practice, but they still sabotage the integrity of research results and, sometimes, the health of human subjects.

Commercial sources of income often distort study results. Northfield Laboratories, the makers of PolyHeme, paid institutions a bounty of $10,000 for each subject *in addition to* the hundreds of thousands of dollars they paid each institution actually to conduct the research. Samuel Tisherman, principal investigator of the University of Maryland's hypothermia experiment, stands to accrue a windfall should his patented hypothermia-research process succeed. When physician-researchers are paid by the pharmaceutical industry, their medical-journal findings exhibit clear bias in line with the interests of the sponsoring company. As I reported in the *American Scholar:*

148   Drs. Paul M. Ridker and Jose Torres at Harvard Medical School found that 67 percent of the results of industry-sponsored trials published between 2000 and 2005 in the three most influential medical publications favored the sponsoring company's experimental heart drugs and often its devices. Trials funded by nonprofits, however, were as likely to support the drugs or devices as to oppose them, and studies that combined industry funding with nonprofit support fell between the two on the spectrum, with 57 percent offering favorable results.

Not all conflicts of interest are financial. Professional advancement, such as academic promotions (with higher salaries), being given laboratories within medical centers, prizes, fame, and even being widely lauded as a medical benefactor are also powerful incentives to cut ethical corners, including abandoning consent.

Because the putative benefits to the subjects are trumpeted by researchers but the significant benefits to the researchers and institutions are ignored, this "benefactor" label is sometimes misapplied. Even exploitative research can be inaccurately valorized as altruistic, beneficial, and "for the common good." IRBs should be tasked with ensuring that the descriptions of research to the public are free of these deceptions (including omissions) and this accuracy should be a condition of IRB approval.

Mandate a Full IRB Review for Every Study
"Expedited review" by an IRB can consist of evaluation by only a single member of the board. This is simply insufficient, especially given the large number of troubled studies that have emerged after IRB review, and should no longer be permitted.

Require a Mandate for Change

Instead of ad hoc waivers, IRBs should be required to ensure that proof of a mandate exists for each "research without consent" study. Ethicist Robert Veatch once suggested that such mandates should approximate 95 percent of the affected community.

The silence with which consent has been insidiously taken off the table is an inexcusable breach of trust. The right to give or withhold consent has been sacred in this country throughout its history. It was U.S. lawyers and doctors who confronted Nazi researchers about robbing their subjects of consent. After Nuremberg, Americans have been repeatedly assured of this right via state and local laws, hospital practice codes, and the Code of Federal Regulations.

Unveil the Process

In 1974, when news reports revealed that Tuskegee farmers as well as prisoners across the U.S. had joined middle-class Americans exposed to radiation and African Americans subjected to centuries of secret nonconsensual research, Americans reacted with unqualified outrage—and laws that restricted prison research and stricter scrutiny of research with vulnerable population.

So, when researchers found it increasingly convenient and profitable to deny consent, they did it quietly. So secretly was the right to consent restricted that, twenty-four years later, most Americans still do not know they have lost this key right and protection.

Some may challenge my characterization of this action as secret, noting that a great deal of discussion took place among researchers, ethicists, IRBs, and university staff. But the fraught discussions as described in Chapter Three took place only among those involved with conducting medical research—which seems not to include the laypersons without whom no research can be performed. The latter alone bear the research's health risks but benefits have rarely accrued to them, only to the researchers and, possibly, to future patients. Because the conversation that resulted in the rollback (and current execution) of consent excluded subjects, this fits Marcel Pagnol's definition: "A secret is not something unrevealed, but told privately in a whisper."

Eschew Newspeak

The honest sharing of information and debate concerning human medical experimentation that must inform any decision about consent is rendered impossible by the corruption of the language and semiotics adopted by researchers, their institutions, and by too many ethics experts.

In December 2017, the science-challenged Trump administration banned seven terms from official use by Centers for Disease Control and Prevention officials: *vulnerable, entitlement, diversity, transgender, fetus, evidence-based*, and *science-based*.

Why? Banning "science-based" speaks for itself, especially when the administration urged substituting language about community standards. The overall intent of this latter-day newspeak is clear, as George Orwell warned in *1984* when he wrote (as I noted earlier), "The purpose of Newspeak was not only to provide a medium of expression for the worldview and mental habits proper to the devotees of INGSOC, but to make all other modes of thought impossible."

Curtailing language limits our ability not only to express thoughts, but also to formulate them. When people who are involuntarily separated from their organs are exclusively referred to as "donors," how does one suggest that a theft has occurred? When the process of being unwittingly coerced into dangerous research is unanimously described by scientists as "emergency treatment," sanctioned by your "community consent," "presumed consent," "deferred consent," or "blanket consent," arguing that you have been forced into a medical experiment becomes a quixotic debate in a hall of semantic fun-house mirrors.

As I note above, EFIC regulations and discussions always refer to dispensing with "informed consent," but it is actually *any* form of consent that is banned. The rationale is that a subject is not conscious or even lucid enough to understand a detailed risk-benefit analysis, but the rule is also withholding simple consent, of which they might be capable.

Community notification was originally referred to as "community consent," although consent is not a feature of the meeting or the research. "Notification" remains inaccurate, given the few in the potential subject pool who have been reached with information. "Community" remains an equally deceptive term for a region demarcated solely for the convenience of the research study, not a genuinely cohesive community, designated as such by its members.

"Patients" are conflated with "subjects," and "treatment" is conflated with experimental modalities to deceive patients into what Jay Katz calls "the therapeutic illusion" that lulls subjects into thinking they are receiving cutting-edge treatment or — as

152   in the case of hypothermia—cutting-edge "suspended animation," when in reality they are being used as subjects—exposed
to novel risks for the benefit of others.

For that matter, being forced into research while too ill to
object is characterized as emergency care with terminology like
"exception from informed consent," or EFIC, which stressed
the "emergency" rationale and conflates emergency treatment with research while hiding the experimental nature of the
interaction.

It bears repeating that the rationale of utilitarianism or
beneficence invoked by research organizations fails to mention the monetary or other benefits accruing to the researchers.
In the case of the many failed research studies this book cites,
researchers emerge as the only beneficiaries of the research.

As I noted earlier, even the term "human medical experimentation" has been purged, shunned in favor of more benign-
sounding euphemisms. Many more semantic manipulations
of research subjects have been used to bar their consent. I discuss these in more detail in "Limning the Semantic Frontier of
Informed Consent" in the *Journal of Law, Medicine, and Ethics*.

Until these semantic manipulations are corrected, nonconsensual studies cannot be discussed accurately with laypersons.

Subjects are sometimes promised that they can withdraw
from the studies into which they are forced, even when withdrawal is impossible because they have already been exposed
to risky experimental substances like PolyHeme, ketamine, or
the anthrax vaccine. Federal law should ban such false prom-
ises, and IRBs should be charged with vigilance in rejecting proposals that make such claims.

Reform the IRB

We've known for some time that IRBs allow too much deeply troubled research to go forward. In early June 1998, a Department of Health and Human Services report concluded that IRB members are subject to conflicts of interest, inadequately trained, and overwhelmed by too many cases.

Since 2006, I have suggested integral changes to IRB composition and function that would increase their ability to protect patients and conform to ethical ideals as well as to the law.

Composition: The Office for Protection from Research Risks (OPRR) requires IRBs to have at least five members, only one of whom need be unaffiliated with the institution. But even the few lay members tend to have loyalties to the home institution, and in any event one or two laypersons facing a group of scientific experts cannot be expected to effectively argue for the interest or concerns of the research subjects. Therefore, I propose that each IRB be composed of equal numbers of scientists and of laypersons drawn from the pool of potential subjects.

Some object that laypersons will be unable to understand enough about scientific experiments to judge their suitability and value, but as a medical communicator, I know this is untrue. I know too many skilled and motivated scientists who routinely convey complex information to many naive subjects, although to do so may require some preparation and effort. So do experienced medical communicators and writers who may find a role as "translators" on reformed IRBs.

Besides, the claim that nuanced medical information cannot be conveyed to laypersons is absurd when one considers that if a project cannot be explained to laypersons in an

154   IRB meeting, how does a researcher propose to explain it to the potential subjects, as he must do by law?

Educate medical-research subjects: The researcher who seeks to enroll a subject is also the person charged with objectively explaining the research, and the U.S. medical research system, in order to satisfy the requirements of informed consent. This creates yet another conflict of interest, because many researchers find it impossible to be completely disinterested and as a result they end up "selling" the study rather than describing it.

This conflict doesn't signal a venal motive on the part of researchers: I think it is simply an illogical division of labor. It is unrealistic to ask a researcher to give an utterly objective assessment of her own research study to a potential subject whose participation is key to that study's success.

Instead, the Office of Research Integrity should take leadership in the education of medical subjects and in the description of research studies. It should design and offer such a course, the cost of which should be underwritten by the pharmaceutical firms whose products are tested on the research subjects, much as these firms currently underwrite 40 percent of the FDA's medical evaluations. The course for prospective research subjects will offer education in the essentials of medical research including the role of government and medical institutions, regulations that protect subjects and what responsibilities subjects and researchers owe each other.

Subjects will be given practical information about how research is conducted, what risks and benefits are inherent in different types of research, what their legal rights and moral responsibilities are, what sort of questions they should ask, and how they can maximize their chances of getting the desired result from any clinical trial they choose to enter.

They will be provided with written information such as telephone numbers of advocates to call with questions or complaints and tips on how to determine whether the researcher has a financial interest in the study or some other type of conflict of interest.

This course should be completed in a week or so and meet in local hospitals as well as online for convenience. The certificate of completion awarded on successfully completing the course would be a prerequisite for enrolling in medical research.

Except for patients whose illness is serious enough to preclude their attendance, only people who have completed this course should be eligible to participate in government-funded clinical trials, and only they should be permitted to serve on IRBs.

If the subject is interested in joining a study, it will be described to him and informed consent will be elicited by a dedicated medical communication specialist, not the study investigator.

There is a precedent of sorts for this sort of government-required course in education. The NIH and the Office of Research Integrity require that U.S. medical researchers complete a course on pertinent laws, ethics, and responsibilities in the ethical and practical conduct of biomedical research. I took the course while a research fellow at Harvard Medical School in 2004 and found it factually invaluable and culturally revealing.

I propose that prospective research subjects be given the same advantage.

I also propose that each IRB include a medical ethicist and, if possible, a medical historian who might provide historical

156   context that can alert members to the historical dangers of military expedience or identify parallels between the ethically troubled research proposals of today and the abuses of yesterday.

Maintain ethical protections abroad: 80 percent of clinical trials by U.S. research organizations are now conducted abroad, far from governmental scrutiny and with a disturbingly casual approach to informed consent. This is disturbing because we cannot retain moral credibility if we champion human rights in medical research at home and ignore them abroad. Researchers should be made to follow informed-consent strictures abroad that are as restrictive as those governing their research on American shores.

The Devil's Advocate/Tenth (Wo)Man: From the laxity that permitted exposing Baltimore children to lead to the greed that caused Coast to approve a risky and fictitious study, too much IRB "scrutiny" of studies could be dismissed as rubber-stamping. Such lapses would be discouraged by the adoption of a "devil's advocate" strategy. In the case of a unanimous or nearly unanimous decision, this would require appointing one member to construct the most compelling case possible against the board's unanimous determination. So, should an entire board vote for approval, the "tenth (wo)man" or devil's advocate would be required to adopt and vigorously support an alternative decision. The hope is that this critique will spur greater nuance in the board's thinking and reveal any flaw—or conflict of interest—in the board's assessment.

Why preserve informed consent in medical research? It helps to shore up autonomy, respect, and justice, which are all essential to the ethical conduct of medicine. However, given the more sordid chapters in the history of U.S. medicine, many people warily view consent as an essential layer of protection against bodily appropriation, not as a philosophical abstraction. When the U.S. covertly withdrew consent, this weakened trust in the medical system, recalling the lament of George Bernard Shaw, who wrote,

> I do not know a single thoughtful and well-informed person who does not feel that the tragedy of illness at present is that it delivers you helplessly into the hands of a profession which you deeply mistrust.

TYPE OF "CONSENT"	DEFINITION	INFORMED? ARE YOU TOLD THE DETAILS?	
Informed consent	Consent that is predicated upon a complete and unbiased presentation of known pertinent facts before, during, and after the research study in question	Yes	
Presumed consent	Assumes subject would consent, so requires dissenters to opt out	No	
Community consent	Description of experimentation to be conducted within subject's area	No	
Consent by proxy	Another person is called on to offer a substitute informed consent	Yes, but only after you are enrolled	
Deferred subject consent	Consent from subject after it has already taken place	Yes, but only after you are enrolled	
Deferred proxy consent	From next of kin after already taken place	No?	
Implied consent	"General" consent applied to discrete studies/procedures	Not for subsequent studies	
Blanket consent (waiver of consent)	Permission to use tissue or information for any purpose	No	
Broad consent	Permission to use tissue or information for a variety of purposes	No	

FAMILY LEGAL REPRESENTATIVE NOTIFIED?	ELICITED BEFORE OR AFTER PROCEDURE?	CAN SUBJECT WITHHOLD HIS/ HER CONSENT?	RATIONALE
Sometimes, particularly if the subject is not a competent adult	Before	Yes	Mandates, including the Nuremberg Code, and the autonomy dictates of the Belmont Report
No	Never	No, unless a convenient, well-publicized opt-out scheme exists	Societal norms in treatment setting; various noninclusive "majority-will" surveys, or no rationale
No	Never	No	Researcher convenience
Yes	Never	No	Alleged societal norms
No	After	No	Researcher convenience
Yes	Never	No	Researcher convenience; alleged societal norms
No	Neither	No	Researcher convenience
No	Before the first study only	Only for the first study	"Generally considered unacceptable"
No	Before the first study only	Only for the first study	Researcher convenience

1.   The voluntary consent of the human subject is absolutely essential. This means that the person involved should have legal capacity to give consent; should be so situated as to be able to exercise free power of choice, without the intervention of any element of force, fraud, deceit, duress, over-reaching, or other ulterior form of constraint or coercion; and should have sufficient knowledge and comprehension of the elements of the subject matter involved, as to enable him to make an understanding and enlightened decision. This latter element requires that, before the acceptance of an affirmative decision by the experimental subject, there should be made known to him the nature, duration, and purpose of the experiment; the method and means by which it is to be conducted; all inconveniences and hazards reasonably to be expected; and the effects upon his health or person, which may possibly come from his participation in the experiment. The duty and responsibility for ascertaining the quality of the consent rests upon each individual who initiates, directs or engages in the experiment. It is a personal duty and responsibility which may not be delegated to another with impunity.

2.   The experiment should be such as to yield fruitful results for the good of society, unprocurable by other methods or means of study, and not random and unnecessary in nature.

3.   The experiment should be so designed and based on the results of animal experimentation and a knowledge of the natural history of the disease or other problem under study, that the anticipated results will justify the performance of the experiment.

4.   The experiment should be so conducted as to avoid all unnecessary physical and mental suffering and injury.

5.   No experiment should be conducted, where there is an a priori reason to believe that death or disabling injury will occur; except, perhaps, in those experiments where the experimental physicians also serve as subjects.

6.   The degree of risk to be taken should never exceed that determined by the humanitarian importance of the problem to be solved by the experiment.

162   7.   Proper preparations should be made and adequate facilities provided
to protect the experimental subject against even remote possibilities of
injury, disability, or death.

8.   The experiment should be conducted only by scientifically qualified
persons. The highest degree of skill and care should be required through all
stages of the experiment of those who conduct or engage in the experiment.

9.   During the course of the experiment, the human subject should be at
liberty to bring the experiment to an end, if he has reached the physical or
mental state, where continuation of the experiment seemed to him to be
impossible.

10.   During the course of the experiment, the scientist in charge must
be prepared to terminate the experiment at any stage, if he has probable
cause to believe, in the exercise of the good faith, superior skill and careful
judgement required of him, that a continuation of the experiment is likely
to result in injury, disability, or death to the experimental subject.

The question of dwindling access to informed consent in U.S. medical research has consumed me since the 1990s, when I held a fellowship at the Harvard School of Public Health. Under the expert guidance of fellowship director Robert Meyers, I was introduced to the work of many groundbreaking scholars like *New England Journal of Medicine* editor Marcia Angell as well as George Annas and Michael Grodin, authors of *The Nazi Doctors and the Nuremberg Code*. They generously shared their time and expertise with me, and when I returned as a Medical Ethics Fellow at the medical school, so did the late Jay Katz of Yale and professor Allan Brandt, author of definitive studies on the "Tuskegee syphilis experiment" and of *The Cigarette Century*.

I am equally grateful to those inspirations who also have been more recently generous with their expertise, resources, and valuable time. These include University of Minnesota professor Carl Elliott, Karla Holloway of Duke University, Northeastern University's Patricia Williams, Nancy King of Duke, Dorothy Roberts of the University of Pennsylvania, and Michele Bratcher Goodwin, professor at the University of California at Irvine, and Yuki Kuromaru.

Portions of this work have appeared elsewhere, and I thank Edward J. Hutchinson, editor of the *Journal of Law, Medicine, and Ethics*, for allowing me to include portions of my essay "Limning the Semantic Frontiers of Informed Consent" from the journal's Fall 2016 issue. I am also grateful to Robert Wilson, editor of *The American Scholar*, which published my essay "The Ethics of Consent" concerning informed-consent restrictions during the coronavirus pandemic in its September 30, 2020 issue Material from my January 2012 article in *New Scientist* entitled "Too many given no right to refuse in medical trials" also appears in this book.

But perhaps I owe the most to Columbia University's Nicholas Lemann, the director of Columbia Global Reports, who I thank for the opportunity to share what I have learned about the insidious decay of informed consent, once the linchpin of ethical U.S. medical research.

I am grateful, as always, for the warmth and keen judgment of my wonderful agent, Lisa Bankoff, and I am thrilled by the opportunity to thank Jimmy So, editor of Columbia Global Reports, for his incisive feedback and organizational genius. I thank Alondra Nelson, Social Science Chair at the Institute for Advanced Study, the *New York Times*'s Sheri L. Fink, Joshua Prager, Randi Hutter Epstein, and Hilda Hutcherson, Associate Dean for Diversity and Minority Affairs at Columbia University Medical Center, as

164   well as Robert Klitzman, chair of the Columbia University bioethics master's program, for their early and constant support.

My fellow scribes of the Invisible Institute, founded by Annie Murphy Paul and Alissa Quart, have proven to be trusted advisers. These pillars of support include Kaja Perina, Susan Cain, Abby Ellin, Tom Zoellner, Wendy Paris, Christine Kenneally, Catherine Orenstein, Katherine Stewart, Elizabeth DeVita-Raeburn, Paul Raeburn, Ron Leiber, Maia Szalavitz, Stacy Sullivan, Gretchen Rubin, Judith Matloff, Lauren Sandler, Ada Calhoun, Gary Bass, Bob Sullivan, and Ron Lieber.

Last but definitely not least, I am blessed in Kate, Eric, and Theresa, my sisters and brother, and I miss Pete every day.

Ron DeBose is always with me.

Harriet A. Washington, *Medical Apartheid: The Dark History of Medical Experimentation on Black Americans from Colonial Times to the Present* (Doubleday, 2008)

Harriet A. Washington, *Deadly Monopolies: The Shocking Corporate Takeover of Life Itself—And the Consequences for Your Health and Our Medical Future* (Doubleday, 2012)

Jay Katz, Alexander Morgan Capron, Eleanor Swift Glass, *Experimentation with Human Beings: The Authority of the Investigator, Subject, Professions, and State in the Human Experimentation Process* (Russell Sage Foundation, 1972)

Osagie K. Obasogie, Marcy Darnovsky, eds., *Beyond Bioethics: Toward a New Biopolitics* (University of California Press, 2018)

Carl Elliott, *White Coat, Black Hat: Adventures on the Dark Side of Medicine* (Beacon Press, 2010)

Dorothy Roberts, *Killing the Black Body: Race, Reproduction, and the Meaning of Liberty* (Vintage, 1998)

Michele Goodwin, *Policing the Womb: Invisible Women and the Criminalization of Motherhood* (Cambridge University Press, 2020)

NOTES

PREFACE

8   **found that nineteen still tested positive:** Nick Powell, "Even After Deaths and Positive Tests, Texas City Doctor Declares Victory with Trump-Touted Drug," *Houston Chronicle*, May 14, 2020. Accessed at https://www.houstonchronicle.com/news/houston-texas/houston/article/texas-city-nursing-home-doc-unproven-trump-drug-15270476.php.

9   **they were "more than prepared" to make hydroxychloroquine available:** "Anti-Malarial Drug to Be Tried on 3,000 COVID-19 Patients in Detroit Hospital: U.S. Vice President TWC India," IANS (India's Independent Newswire), April 6, 2020. Accessed at https://weather.com/en-IN/india/coronavirus/news/2020-04-06-anti-malarial-drug-trial-against-covid-19-to-be-used-in-detroit.

9   **prescriptions for hydroxychloroquine spiked by 367 percent:** Tori Marsh, "Live Updates: Fills and Prices for Unproven COVID-19 Treatments," GoodRx, June 16, 2020. Accessed at https://www.goodrx.com/blog/covid-19-treatments-fill-increases-price-changes/.

10   **"If I had to call all the families for every medicine that I started on a patient":** Nick Powell and

Taylor Goldenstein, "Treatment of COVID-19 Patients at Texas City Nursing Home Draws Ethical Questions," *Houston Chronicle*, April 10, 2020 (updated April 13, 2020).

10   **it does not present an excuse for abandoning ethical behavior:** "How Far Is too Far in Coronavirus Fight? Texas City Nursing Home Doctor Crosses Ethical Line," *Texan*, April 15, 2020.

10   **cut short when subjects developed irregular heartbeats:** Mayla Gabriela Silva Borba, Fernando Fonseca Almeida Val, Vanderson Souza Sampeio, et al, "Chloroquine Diphosphate in Two Different Dosages as Adjunctive Therapy of Hospitalized Patients with Severe Respiratory Syndrome in the Context of Coronavirus (SARS-CoV-2) Infection: Preliminary Safety Results of a Randomized, Double-Blinded, Phase IIb Clinical Trial (CloroCovid-19 Study)," *JAMA Network Open*, April 24, 2020. doi: 10.1001/jamanetworkopen.2020.8857.

10   **"recent data from a large randomized controlled trial showed no evidence of benefit":** "Letter to Gary Disbrow, PhD., Deputy Assistant Secretary Director, Medical Countermeasure Programs, BARDA," Food and Drug Administration, June 15, 2020. Accessed at https://www.fda.gov/media/138945/download.

168   13   **declared these victims dead at the scene:** Rukmini Callimachi, "Paramedics, Strained in the Hot Zone, Pull Back From CPR," *New York Times*, May 19, 2020.

14   **from forty minutes to about ten minutes:** Rukmini Callimachi, "Paramedics, Strained in the Hot Zone, Pull Back From CPR."

15   **people with physical or mental disabilities were ordered murdered:** Matt Lebovic "80 Years Ago, Lethal Nazi T4 Center Began Euthanizing Germans with Disabilities," *Times of Israel,* May 9, 2020.

16   **to withdraw ventilators from the elderly and the disabled:** Clare Wilson, "End-of-Life Medical Decisions Being Rushed Through Due to Coronavirus," *New Scientist*, April 17, 2020. Accessed at https://www.newscientist.com/article/2240401-end-of-life-medical-decisions-being-rushed-through-due-to-coronavirus/.

17   **treating people who are younger and healthier:** Carol Marbin Miller, "Civil Rights Leaders to DeSantis: Don't Allow States to Withhold Care from the Disabled," *Miami Herald*, April 2, 2020. Accessed at https://www.miamiherald.com/news/coronavirus/article241676431.html.

18   **"it is ethically appropriate for physicians to withdraw it":** "Withholding or Withdrawing Life-Sustaining Treatment," *AMA Principles of Medical Ethics: I, III, IV, V*, November 14, 2016, *Code of Medical Ethics Opinion* 5.3. Accessed at https://www.ama-assn.org/delivering-care/ethics/withholding-or-withdrawing-life-sustaining-treatment.

18   **The U.S. courts have supported this:** Clarence H. Braddock III, MD, MPH, "Termination of Life-Sustaining Treatment," University of Washington Medicine Department of Bioethics and Humanities. Accessed at http://depts.washington.edu/bhdept/ethics-medicine/bioethics-topics/articles/termination-life-sustaining-treatment.

18   **should not receive ventilation if they were classified as "frail":** Clare Wilson, "End-of-life Medical Decisions Being Rushed Through Due to Coronavirus."

20   **I had seen this very suggestion proposed and discussed:** Michael Pauron, "Harriet A. Washington: L'Afrique est le laboratoire de l'Occident," *Mondafrique*, April 10, 2020. Accessed at https://mondafrique.com/author/la-redaction-de-mondafrique/.

20   **relies on scientists' assurance that they have conducted research legally and ethically:** Bethany

Spielman, "Nonconsensual Clinical Trials: A Foreseeable Risk of Offshoring Under Teleglobal Corporatism," *Journal of Bioetheical Inquiry* 12, no. 1 (2015):101–106. doi: 10.1007/s11673-014-9596-2.

21 **who have intentionally administered deadly agents:** Harriet A. Washington "Why Africa Fears Western Medicine," *New York Times,* July 31, 2007. Accessed at https://www .nytimes.com/2007/07/31 /opinion/31washington.html.

21 **infection as a neglected risk factor:** Harriet A. Washington, "The Well Curve: Tropical Diseases Are Undermining Intellectual Development in Countries with Poor Health Care—And They're Coming Here Next," *American Scholar,* September 7, 2015. Accessed at https:// theamericanscholar.org/the -well-curve/#.XtaTQ8Z7k1A.

22 **followed by waves of mental disease and cognition loss:** Harriet A. Washington, *Infectious Madness: The Surprising Science of How We "Catch" Mental Illness* (Little, Brown Spark, 2019).

22 **one in five known cases suffers delirium:** Emily A. Troyer, "Are We Facing a Crashing Wave of Neuropsychiatric Sequelae of COVID-19? Neuropsychiatric Symptoms and Potential Immunologic Mechanisms," *Brain, Behavior, and Immunity,*

April 13, 2020. doi: 10.1016/j. bbi.2020.04.027.

22 **neurologic problems haunted 78 of 214 patients:** A. M. Franceschi, "Hemorrhagic Posterior Reversible Encephalopathy Syndrome as a Manifestation of COVID-19 Infection," *American Journal of Neuroradiology,* May 2020. doi: 10.3174/ajnr.A6595.

22 **Strokes, which cause cognitive losses of memory:** T. M. Leslie-Mazwi, et al, "Preserving Access: A Review of Stroke Thrombectomy During the COVID-19 Pandemic," *American Journal of Neuroradiology,* May 21, 2020. doi: 10.3174/ajnr.A6606.

22–23 **a dramatic increase from their preinfection prevalence:** Emily A. Troyer, "Are We Facing a Crashing Wave of Neuropsychiatric Sequelae of COVID-19?"

CHAPTER ONE

24 **Private First Class Jemekia Barber:** She has remarried and now uses the surname Weeden. In this text I have used the surname cited in the news accounts and lawsuits to which I refer.

24 **as I read:** *Jemekia Barber v. the United States of America Jemekia Barber v. United States Army* No. 03-1056 (D.C. No. 00-N-1022 (MJW)) (District of Colorado), filed December 2003, U.S. Court of Appeals, Tenth Circuit.

170   25   **She refused to take a six-shot series of experimental anthrax vaccinations:** In 1990, the Department of Defense (DOD) sought and obtained from the Food and Drug Administration a waiver of the informed-consent requirements for human medical experimentation. Under Rule 21 CFR 50.23(d), soldiers suddenly lost the protection of the informed-consent provisions that give other Americans the right to say no. *Medical Apartheid*, p. 398. See also George J. Annas, "Protecting Soldiers from Friendly Fire: The Consent Requirement for Using Investigational Drugs and Vaccines in Combat," *American Journal of Law and Medicine* (Summer–Fall 1998), p. 53.

25   **She disobeyed that order on the ground:** *Jemekia Barber v. United States Army* No. 03-1056 (D.C. No. 00-N-1022 (MJW)) (District of Colorado) filed December 2003, U.S. Court of Appeals Tenth Circuit.

27   **but Blacks were overrepresented:** Defense Equal Opportunity Management Institute (DEOMI)).

27   **"The side effects I read about were alarming":** "Vaccine Refuser Court-Martialed," CBS News, May 28, 2003. Accessed at https://www.cbsnews.com/news/vaccine-refuser-court-martialed/.

27   **at least four hundred soldiers had been disciplined:** Laura Rozen, "The Anthrax Vaccine Scandal: Why Did the Pentagon Allow Bioport Corp. to Remain the Sole U.S. Supplier of a Crucial Weapon Against Bioterror, Despite Years of Failure to Deliver the Vaccine?" *Salon,* October 15, 2001. Accessed at https://www.salon.com/2001/10/15/anthrax_vaccine/.

27   **It attributed complaints to "emotional issues":** Laura Rozen, "The Anthrax Vaccine Scandal."

28   **This version of sovereign immunity arose from a trio of unsuccessful 1950 suits:** In *Feres v. United States,* 340 U.S. 135 (1950), the U.S. Supreme Court ruled that the United States is not liable under the Federal Tort Claims Act for injuries to members of the armed forces sustained while on active duty and not on furlough and resulting from the negligence of others in the armed forces. The opinion is an extension of the English common-law concept of sovereign immunity.

29   **anthrax is characterized by a constellation of flu-like symptoms:** "Anthrax Symptoms and Causes," Mayo Clinic. Accessed at https://www.mayoclinic.org/diseases-conditions/anthrax/symptoms-causes/syc-20356203.

29   **the Greek word for charcoal:** "Charcoal: ξυλάνθρακας," *In Different Languages* (IDL). Accessed at https://www.indifferentlanguages.com/words/charcoal/greek/edit.

29   or most dangerously, through inhalation: John R. Barra, Anne E. Boyera, and Conrad P. Quinna, "Anthrax: Modern Exposure Science Combats a Deadly, Ancient Disease," *Exposure Science Digest*, U.S. Centers for Disease Control and Prevention. doi:10.1038 /jes.2010.4,

30   South Africa, for example, unleashed it against Zimbabwe: Gavin Cameron, Jason Pate, and Kathleen M. Vogel, "Planting Fear: How Real Is the Threat of Agricultural Terrorism?" *Bulletin of the Atomic Scientists* 57, no. 5 (2001), pp. 38–44.

30   allows the DOD to experiment on service personnel without their consent or knowledge: It "permits drug-by-drug waiver approval" on the basis that consent is "not feasible" in a "specific military operation involving combat or the immediate threat of combat." George J. Annas, "Protecting Soldiers from Friendly Fire," p. 349.

31   just four decades after the Army oversaw the Nuremberg trial: Harriet A. Washington, "Untrue Blood," unpublished manuscript, 2009.

31   the Edgewood Arsenal human experiments: Morgan Knibbe, "The Atomic-Bomb Guinea Pigs: U.S. Veterans Break the Forced Silence," *Atlantic*, May 27, 2019. Accessed at

https://www.theatlantic.com/video /index/590299/atomic-soldiers/.

32   a Japanese doomsday cult: Holly Fletcher, "Aum Shinrikyo: A Profile of the Japanese Religious Cult That Carried Out the 1995 Subway Sarin Attack," Council on *Foreign Relations*, June 19, 2012. Accessed at https://www.cfr.org /backgrounder/aum-shinrikyo.

32   alleged that at least ten nations were then developing: Letter from William Cohen, Secretary of Defense, to Representative Christopher Shays et al, U.S. House of Representatives, September 30, 1999, quoted in *Fourth Report by the Committee on Government Reform Together with Dissenting and Supplemental Views*, "The Department of Defense Anthrax Vaccine Immunization Program: Unproven Force Protection, H.R. Doc. NO. 106-556, at 18" (2000). Accessed at http:// www.house.gov/reform/ns/reports /anthraxreport.pdf.

32   twenty-six Senate staffers and five police officers were exposed: John Lancaster and Susan Schmidt, "Exposed to Anthrax on Capitol Hill," *Washington Post*, October 18, 2001.

32   which processed letters contaminated with anthrax, did not close: Marilyn W. Thompson, "Survivor, Brentwood; Leroy Richmond Was Hit with a Biological Weapon in the Line of

172   Duty. His Experience Just Might Be Instructive," *Washington Post Magazine,* March 30, 2003, p. W18; See also Shankar Vedantam and Mary Pat Flaherty, "CDC Rushed Paperwork for Anthrax Vaccinations; 48 Congressional Aides Received Inoculations," *Washington Post,* December 22, 2001, p. 10.

33   **postal workers complained that they feared contamination:** These were followed by more recent efforts to bomb New York's Lincoln Tunnel and a plot—foiled in July 2002—for a rush-hour bombing of a Brooklyn subway station.

33   **Mortality during the anthrax-letter attacks:** Daniel B. Jernigan, et al, "Investigation of Bioterrorism-Related Anthrax, United States, 2001: Epidemiologic Findings," *Emerging Infectious Diseases,* Volume 8, Number 10—October 2002.

33   **anthrax vaccine production was in crisis, too:** Laura Rozen, "The Anthrax Vaccine Scandal."

33   **soldiers began complaining of side effects:** Laura Rozen, "The Anthrax Vaccine Scandal."

33   **about 570,000 military personnel had received at least one shot:** Michael Kilian, "Lawmakers Hit Military on Anthrax Vaccination," *Chicago Tribune,* June 1, 2000.

33   **more than 400 "refusers" had been disciplined for insubordination:** Benjamin Krause, "Leaked Anthrax Vaccine Memo Likely Authentic," Disabled Veterans, April 17, 2018. Accessed at https://www.disabledveterans .org/2018/04/17/leaked-anthrax -vaccine- memo-likely-authentic/.

34   **Dingle determined that the vaccine was unsafe and ineffective:** Thomas D. Williams, "Vaccine Policy," *Hartford Courant,* September 9, 2005.

36   **"The commander believed that characterization was warranted":** *Jemekia Barber, v. United States Army,* No. 03-1056 (District of Colorado) filed December 2003, U.S. Court of Appeals, Tenth Circuit.

37   **Yet in 2001 Buck was court-martialed:** Mark Thompson, "The Buck Stops (the Anthrax Shots) Here," *Time,* January 12, 2001.

37   **wrote to members of Congress asking them to intervene:** Thomas D. Williams, "R. Dingle Dies; Fought Anthrax-Vaccine Policy," *Hartford Courant,* September 9, 2005.

37   **He was sentenced to sixty days of base restriction:** "Air Force Physician Convicted of Disobeying Order in Anthrax Vaccine Case," Associated Press, May 21, 2001. Accessed at https://www.foxnews .com/story/air-force-physician

-convicted-of-disobeying-order
-in-anthrax-vaccine-case.

38   **"Well, I think that's a part
of what you do when you raise
your right hand"**: The author's
telephone conversations with
Leernest Ruffin on May 24, 2019,
and September 3, 2019.

39   **ordered the government to
"turn the plane around"**: Suzanne
Gamboa and Jacob Soboroff, "Judge
Orders Plane Carrying Deported
Mother and Child Turned Around,
Blocks More Removals," NBC
News, August 9, 2018. Accessed at
https://www.nbcnews.com
/storyline/immigration-border
-crisis/judge-orders-plane
-carrying-deported-mother-child
-turned-around-blocks-n899311.

39   **members of the armed forces
also serve as guinea pigs**: George
A. Jelinek, "Time for change,"
Emergency Medicine, Nov. 3, 2003,
p. 348.

40   **belatedly admitted that
vaccinations had harmed some
troops badly**: Patrick Steven
McGrath, "Subject: Tasking
Order 18-04-01 (Soldier Anthrax
Vaccination 2001–2007),"
Department of Defense, 2nd
Battalion, 1st Air Defense Artillery
Regiment, 35th Air Defense
Artillery Brigade, Unit #15754,
April 10, 2018.

40   **the DOD had dismissed the
leaked document as a "fake" and a**

"scam": Benjamin Krause, "Leaked
Anthrax Vaccine Memo Likely
Authentic."

40   **an independent legal
analysis determined the memo:**
Benjamin Krause, "Leaked
Anthrax Vaccine Memo Likely
Authentic."

40   **an FBI investigation that
had spanned eight years and six
continents**: Joby Warrick, "FBI
Investigation of 2001 Anthrax
Attacks Concluded; U.S. Releases
Details," *Washington Post*, February
20, 2010. Accessed at http://
www.washingtonpost.com/wp
-dyn/content/article/2010/02/19
/AR2010021902369.html.

41   **"the worst act of bioterrorism
in U.S. history"**: Joby Warrick,
"FBI Investigation of 2001 Anthrax
Attacks Concluded; U.S. Releases
Details."

41   **out of concern for the
future of an anthrax vaccination
program**: Rachel Swarns and Eric
Lipton, "From a Helper to the
Suspect in the Anthrax Case," *New
York Times*, August 7, 2008.

42   **there exists no legal decision
to definitively establish his guilt:**
Stephen Engelberg, "New Evidence
Adds Doubt to FBI's Case Against
Anthrax Suspect," Pro Publica,
October 10, 2011. Accessed at
https://www.propublica.org
/article/new-evidence-disputes
-case-against-bruce-e-ivins.

174   42   **By a conservative estimate, 2,500 soldiers refused:** Harriet A. Washington, "Untrue Blood."

42   **surveyed 829 Air Force pilots:** At the time there were 176,000 troops in the Guard and Reserve, including about 13,000 who are pilots or other air crew members. Jamie McIntyre, "Congressional Report says Anthrax Vaccine Large Part of Air Force Exodus," CNN. com, October 11, 2000. Accessed at https://www.cnn.com/2000 /US/10/11/anthrax.military/.

42   **concerns about the safety of the mandatory shots played a role:** Jamie McIntyre, "Congressional Report Says Anthrax Vaccine Large Part of Air Force Exodus."

CHAPTER TWO

43   **the Nuremberg Code, a set of ethical guidelines for human experimentation:** George J. Annas and Michael Grodin (eds.), *The Nazi Doctors and the Nuremberg Code: Human Rights in Human Experimentation* (Oxford University Press, 1995), p. 3.

44   **Nazi experiments conducted on Jews, Poles, Afro-Germans:** Clarence Lusane, *Hitler's Black Victims* (Routledge, 2000), pp. 139–140; see also Robert W. Kesting, "Blacks Under the Swastika: A Research Note," *Journal of Negro History* 83, no. 1 (1998), pp. 84–99 and *"Reichsministerium des Innern,"* archives, the U.S. Holocaust Memorial Museum (June 19, 1937).

44   **U.S. Atomic Energy Commission issued a memo that advocated for stringent informed consent:** Dan Guttman, "Human Radiation Experiments: The Still Unfolding Legacy," *Civil Rights Journal* (Fall 2000), pp. 30–31.

44   **subjected others to limb amputations without anesthesia:** *Nuremberg Military Tribunals, Trials of War Criminals, Under Council Control Law No. 10,* Nuremberg, October 1946–April 1949, vol. 2 (Washington, D.C.: U.S. Government Printing Office, 1949).

44   **researchers invoked the need to urgently address the soldiers' welfare:** George J. Annas and Michael Grodin, *The Nazi Doctors and the Nuremberg Code*, pp. 20, 23, 174–182.

45   **U.S. federal consent principles were very inconsistently applied and rarely formally written:** George J. Annas, "Protecting Soldiers from Friendly Fire: The Consent Requirement for Using Investigational Drugs and Vaccines in Combat," *American Journal of Law & Medicine* 24, no. 2/3 (January 1, 1998).

45   **the less constricting World Medical Association's Code of Ethics:** "World Medical Association Code of Ethics," *British Medical Journal* 1119 (1962).

46 **Eugenics was applied:** Harriet A. Washington, *Medical Apartheid: The Dark History of Medical Experimentation on Black Americans from Colonial Times to the Present* (Doubleday, 2007), p. 190.

47 **doctors invented racial hygiene:** George J. Annas and Michael Grodin, *The Nazi Doctors and the Nuremberg Code*, pp. 17, 19.

48 **describing the U.S. Army wartime experiments on eight hundred prisoners:** "Prison Malaria: Convicts Expose Themselves to Disease So Doctors Can Study It," *Life*, June 4, 1945, pp. 43–46.

48 **at the Stateville Penitentiary near Joliet, Illinois:** Jay Katz and Alexander Capron, *Experimentation with Human Beings: The Authority of the Investigator, Subject, Professions, and State in the Human Experimentation Process* (Russell Sage Foundation, 1972).

48 **they were administered untested drugs under controlled conditions:** Franklin G. Miller, "The Stateville Penitentiary Malaria Experiments: A Case Study in Retrospective Ethical Assessment," *Perspectives in Biology and Medicine* 56, no. 4, pp. 548–567. doi:10.1353/pbm.2013.0035.

49 **an opportunity to craft a global standard for research ethics and human rights:** George J. Annas and Michael Grodin, *The Nazi Doctors and the Nuremberg Code*, p. 3.

49 **has come to ignore Nuremberg's uncompromising insistence on informed consent:** Rebecca S. Holmes-Farley and Michael A Grodin. "Foreword: Law, Medicine and Socially Responsible Research," *American Journal of Law & Medicine* 24, no. 2/3 (January 1, 1998).

CHAPTER THREE

53 **welcomed Carlos:** His name has been changed to preserve his privacy.

54 **I was conscious while an EMT gave me blood:** Martha was given not blood, but the artificial blood substitute PolyHeme, which is red and resembles blood.

58 **has been one of the most aggressive supporters of HBOC research:** Dr. Steven Galvan, "U.S. Army Institute of Surgical Research Celebrates 70th Anniversary," Joint Base San Antonio Links, August 13, 2018. Accessed at https://www.jbsa.mil/News/News/Article/1600643/us-army-institute-of-surgical-research-celebrates-70th-anniversary/. Dr. Holcomb is now a medical consultant for CellPhire, a Maryland biotechnology company whose products include a freeze-dried blood product for trauma care.

58   **Holcomb is now a medical consultant for CellPhire:** John B. Holcomb, M.D., F.A.C.S., Joins Cellphire as Medical Consultant," Cellphire press release, May 15, 2019. Accessed at https://www.cellphire.com/john-holcomb/–.

58   **"strongly advocates conducting clinical trials to improve trauma care":** C. James Carrico, John B. Holcomb, Irshad H. Chaudry, "Scientific Priorities and Strategic Planning for Resuscitation Research and Life Saving Therapy Following Traumatic Injury: Report of the PULSE Trauma Work Group. Post Resuscitative and Initial Utility of Life Saving Efforts," *Shock* 17 (2002), pp. 165–168. doi: 10.1111/j.1553-2712.2002.tb02303.x; Alex Berenson, "Army's Aggressive Surgeon Is Too Aggressive for Some," *New York Times,* November 6, 2007. Accessed at https://www.nytimes.com/2007/11/06/health/06prof.html.

58   **Its results were disastrous:** Thomas M. Burton, "Amid Alarm Bells, a Blood Substitute Keeps Pumping," *Wall Street Journal,* February 22, 2006. Accessed at https://www.wsj.com/articles/SB114057765651379801; also see Alex Berenson, "Army's Aggressive Surgeon Is Too Aggressive for Some."

58   **"he should never have approved the trial for his center":** Alex Berenson, "Army's Aggressive Surgeon Is Too Aggressive for Some."

59   **"pushed military surgeons to use Factor VII despite a lack of data on its benefits":** Alex Berenson, "Army's Aggressive Surgeon Is Too Aggressive for Some."

59   **which total over 50,000 injuries from hostile fire in Iraq and Afghanistan alone:** "Casualty Status as of 10:00 a.m. EDT Aug. 27, 2019," U.S. Department of Defense. Accessed at https://web.archive.org/web/20130116062321/http://www.defense.gov/news/casualty.pdf.

60   **nearly half of the fifty-two trauma patients infused with it died:** 46 percent.

61   **blood products made up 1.9 percent of all American exports:** Zoe Greenberg, "What Is the Blood of a Poor Person Worth?" *New York Times,* February 1, 2019.

61   **that money can occlude medical judgment and hobble FDA independence:** Harriet A. Washington, *Deadly Monopolies;* "Flacking for Big Pharma," *American Scholar,* Autumn, 2011. "A 2007 paper in the *Public Library of Science* analyzed nearly 200 published comparison trials and found that when a drug is shown to be superior, the study is 20 times more likely to have been funded

by its manufacturer. Positive drug assessments in papers are about 35 times more likely to have been paid for by the drug's maker."

62   **Gould took Northfield public in 1994:** "Memorandum Opinion and Order," Judge George M. Marovich, United States District Court, Northern District Of Illinois, Eastern Division, in Re: Northfield Laboratories, Inc. No. 06 C 1493 Securities Litigation, p. 2.

64   **When involuntary experiments with soldiers was banned:** Jelinek, 2003, p. 348.

64   **although defense appropriations for PolyHeme totaled $4.9 million by mid-2006:** "Despite Northfield's Widening 3Q loss, PolyHeme Trial Progresses," *Medical Device Daily*, April 12, 2006.

65   **fifteen of the sixteen subjects:** All sixteen were subjects, but they were not all infused with PolyHeme: Six were infused with saline, as controls.

65   **ambulances carry PolyHeme:** Eleven of thirty-two, or 34.4 percent.

66   **"the experiment is targeted at several neighborhoods south of I-8":** Matt Potter, "Bad Blood?" *San Diego Reader,* Thursday, July 28, 2005. Porter cited a memo dated August 10, 2004, in which San Diego Emergency Medical Program director Donna Goldsmith wrote that the three

poor communities of Oak Park, Nestor, and San Ysidro were selected because they were the sites of the largest number of severe trauma patients. Goldsmith recorded the expectation that San Diego would ultimately contribute forty PolyHeme subjects.

66   **a bioethicist at the Wake Forest University:** Ken Kipnis, Nancy M. P. King, and Robert M. Nelson, "An Open Letter to Institutional Review Boards Considering Northfield Laboratories' PolyHeme® Trial," *American Journal of Bioethics* 6, no. 3 (2006), pp. 18–21. doi: 10.1080/15265160600685580.

67   **medical condition and time constraints must preclude eliciting informed consent:** There is, of course, another option: One could behave as if one had to experiment to worry about and focus on the person, simply providing that person with the best proven treatment—the standard of care.

69   **those who did appear at "community-notification" meetings:** Jeanne Lenzer, "Blood Not-So-Simple: Should Unconsenting Civilians Be Used in Tests for a Blood Substitute?" *American Prospect,* June, 2006, p. 11.

74   **"The purpose of Newspeak was not only to provide a medium of expression":** George Orwell,

178 "Appendix: The Principles of Newspeak," in *1984*, Project Gutenberg of Australia eBook No. 0100021.txt, 2001. Accessed at http://gutenberg.net.au/ebooks01 /0100021.txt (last visited July 15, 2016).

75 **government-required consent and permission forms were forged or postdated:** "Abdullahi v. Pfizer, Inc." Accessed at https://en.wikipedia.org/wiki /Abdullahi_v._Pfizer,_Inc.

77 **survey results from a limited group of nonconsensual experiments:** William B. Feldman, Spencer P. Hey, and Aaron S. Kesselheim, "Public Approval of Exception from Informed Consent in Emergency Clinical Trials," *JAMA Network Open* 2, no. 7 (July, 2019), p. e197591. Accessed at https://www .ncbi.nlm.nih.gov/pmc/articles /PMC6659147/?report=.

78 **the FDA has granted permission for more than forty:** William B. Feldman, Spencer P. Hey, and Aaron S. Kesselheim, "Public Approval of Exception from Informed Consent in Emergency Clinical Trials."

78 **meaning that they were twice as likely to be conscripted into medical experimentation:** William B. Feldman, Spencer P. Hey, and Aaron S. Kesselheim, "Public Approval of Exception from Informed Consent in Emergency Clinical Trials."

78 **so the number of African Americans could be much higher:** William B. Feldman, Spencer P. Hey, and Aaron S. Kesselheim, "Public Approval of Exception from Informed Consent in Emergency Clinical Trials."

78 **"All trials granted an EFIC must submit documentation of compliance":** William B. Feldman, Spencer P. Hey, and Aaron S. Kesselheim, "Public Approval of Exception from Informed Consent in Emergency Clinical Trials."

CHAPTER FOUR

81 **forced many Americans into studies that violated their right to consent:** Harriet A. Washington, "Too Many Given No Right to Refuse in Medical Trials," *New Scientist,* January 18, 2012. Accessed at https://www.newscientist.com /article/mg21328480-200-too -many-given-no-right-to-refuse -in-medical-trials/.

83 **Dr. T. Stillman placed an advertisement in the *Charleston Mercury*:** Harriet A. Washington, *Medical Apartheid,* p. 133.

83 **to undergo repeated experimental genital surgeries:** Harriet A. Washington, *Medical Apartheid,* p. 64.

83 **were maintained in an infected state, tracked, studied, and ultimately autopsied:** Benjamin Roy, MD, "The Tuskegee

Syphilis Experiment: Medical Ethics, Constitutionalism, and Property in the Body," *Harvard Journal of Minority Public Health* 1, no. 1 (1995), pp. 11–15; James Jones and The Tuskegee Institute, *Bad Blood*, p. 124.

85 **fed the radioactive elements strontium and cesium:** Harriet A. Washington, *Medical Apartheid*, p. 233.

86 **Military physician Joseph Howland injected Ebb Cade:** Harriet A. Washington, *Medical Apartheid*, p. 216.

86 **the Judicial Council of the American Medical Association:** Harriet A. Washington, *Medical Apartheid*, p. 216.

87 **"It's not long since we got through trying Germans for doing exactly the same thing":** Harriet A. Washington, *Medical Apartheid*, p. 218.

87 **"We considered doing such experiments at one time":** Harriet A. Washington, *Medical Apartheid*, p. 218.

88 **most ordinary people were willing to administer:** Adam Cohen, "Four Decades After Milgram, We're Still Willing to Inflict Pain," *New York Times*, December, 28, 2008. Accessed at https://www.nytimes.com /2008/12/29/opinion/29mon3 .html.

88 **Jerry Burger of Santa Clara University replicated the experiment:** Adam Cohen, "Four Decades After Milgram, We're Still Willing to Inflict Pain."

88 **"a remarkable experimental system that blurred the lines":** Nathaniel Comfort, "The Prisoner as Model Organism: Malaria Research at Stateville Penitentiary," *Studies in the History and Philosophy of Biolological Biomedical Science* 40, no. 3 (September 2009), pp. 190–203. doi: 10.1016/j. shpsc.2009.06.007.

89 **steered penniless inmates to research studies:** Harriet A. Washington, *Medical Apartheid*, p. 262.

90 **incarcerated men described time in the research laboratory as a respite for the psyche:** Harriet A. Washington, *Medical Apartheid*, p. 274.

90 **for the first time in their lives find themselves in the role of important human beings:** Hornblum, *Acres of Skin*, p. 65. Reproduced in Harriet A. Washington, *Medical Apartheid*, pp. 262–263.

92 **Harvard researcher Dr. Francis D. Moore wrote:** Jay Katz and Alexander Capron, *Experimentation with Human Beings*, p. 313.

94 **widespread outrage ensued and the program never got off the**

180   **ground:** Michael Reilly, "Organ Ambulances in New York Wait for Dead Bodies to Dismember," *Gizmodo,* June 8, 2008. Accessed at https://i09.gizmodo.com/organ -ambulances-in-new-york-wait -for-dead-bodies-to-di-395488; "NY Introduces Ambulance for Rapid Organ Recovery," *Talk of the Nation,* NPR, May 13, 2008. Accessed at https://www.npr.org /templates/story/story.php?storyId =90404269; Author's telephone interview with Lewis Goldfrank, MD, October 17, 2008.

95   **as described in Michele Bratcher Goodwin's book:** Michele Bratcher Goodwin, *Black Markets: The Supply and Demand of Body Parts* (Cambridge University Press, 2006).

95   **presumed consent alone doesn't drive the variation in organ donation rates:** A Rithalia, C McDaid, S Suekarran, et al, "A Systematic Review of Presumed Consent Systems for Deceased Organ Donation," in *NIHR Health Technology Assessment Programme: Executive Summaries* (Southampton, UK: NIHR Journals Library, 2009). Accessed at https://www.ncbi.nlm .nih.gov/books/NBK56888/.

96   **African American organ and tissue donation:** Thomas Hargrove and Lee Bowman Scripps, "Autopsy Rates Differ by Race, Age, Sex, Education," Howard News Service, August 12, 2009. Accessed at http://www.scrippsnews .com/catego y/author/-thomas -hargrove-and-lee-bowman -scripps-howard-news-service (accessed July 11, 2011). "When looking at all 4.9 million deaths, whites were autopsied less than 6 percent of the time compared to 11 percent for Blacks, 14 percent for Hispanics, 8 percent for Asians and 13 percent for American Indians."

96   **the long history of African-American body appropriation:** Harriet A. Washington, "Vital Signs: Harvesting Organs from Silence," *Emerge Magazine,* January 31, 1995; Janice Frink Brown, "D.C. Gift Act Allows Hospitals to Remove Organs of Crime Victims," *Washington Afro-American,* June 17, 1995.

97   **they fall prey to presumed consent:** Harriet A. Washington, "Vital Signs: Harvesting Organs from Silence," *Emerge Magazine,* January 31, 1995; Janice Frink Brown, "D.C. Gift Act Allows Hospitals to Remove Organs of Crime Victims," *Washington Afro-American,* June 17, 1995.

97   **Even after death, these bodies served pedagogical purposes:** Harriet A. Washington, *Medical Apartheid,* pp. 101–142.

98   **others invoke an individual's moral responsibility to participate in research:** Author's telephone interview with Russell Gruen, July 11, 2009.

99   **given a code number that would enable them to report:** Carl Elliott, "Guinea-pigging: Healthy Human Subjects for Drug-Safety Trials Are in Demand. But Is It a Living?" *New Yorker,* December 30, 2007. Accessed at https://www.newyorker. com/magazine/2008/01/07/ guinea-pigging.

CHAPTER FIVE

100   **Brain activity slows dramatically as the pupils dilate:** Charles Patrick Davis, MD, PhD, "What Are the Symptoms of Hypothermia?" emedicinehealth. Accessed at https://www. emedicinehealth.com/ hypothermia/article_em.htm.

101   **These events make a patient's resuscitation increasingly unlikely:** Nicola Twilley, "Can Hypothermia Save Gunshot Victims?" *New Yorker,* November 28, 2016. Accessed at https://www.newyorker.com /magazine/2016/11/28/can -hypothermia-save-gunshot -victims.

102   **vaguely implies that it is because they suffer high rates of firearms deaths:** Nicola Twilley, "Can Hypothermia Save Gunshot Victims?"

102   **most of these deaths are in white men:** Julia Lurie, "What Kills More Americans: Guns or Cars?" *Mother Jones,* December 14,

2014. Accessed at https://www .motherjones.com/politics/2014/12 /gun-violence-car-deaths-charts/.

102   **nine thousand white men died from firearms in 2012:** Julia Lurie, "What Kills More Americans: Guns or Cars?"

102   **unarmed Black Americans were five times as likely:** Wesley Lowery, "Aren't More White People than Black People Killed by Police? Yes, but No," *Washington Post,* July 11, 2016. Accessed at https://www.washingtonpost .com/news/post-nation/wp /2016/07/11/arent-more-white -people-than-black-people-killed -by-police-yes-but-no/.

103   **university media officer Lisa Clough admitted:** The author's telephone interview with Lisa Clough, February 24, 2020.

103   **did not respond to my repeated email and telephone requests to discuss this work:** Body Cooling Study: Emergency Preservation and Resuscitation for Cardiac Arrest from Trauma (EPR-CAT). Accessed at https:// www.umms.org/ummc/health -services/shock-trauma/news /body-cooling-study.

103   **he optimistically described the research:** Helen Thomson, "Humans Placed in Suspended Animation for the First Time," *New Scientist,* November 20, 2019. Accessed

182   at https://www.newscientist.com
/article/2224004-exclusive
-humans-placed-in-suspended
-animation-for-the-first-time/.

105   "One of my most
fundamental objections to
the regulation is this": J. Katz,
"Blurring the Lines: Research,
Therapy, and IRBs," *Hastings Center
Report* 27, no. 1 (1997), pp. 9–11.
Accessed at http:// www.jstor.org
/stable/3528019.

105   centuries of well-
documented medical abuse
and exploitation: Harriet A.
Washington, *Medical Apartheid*;
J. Walter Fisher, "Physicians and
Slavery in the Antebellum Southern
Medical Journal," *Journal of the
History of Medicine and Allied
Sciences* XXIII (January 1968), p. 45;
"Surgery and the Negro Physician:
Some Parallels in Background,"
National Medical Association Journal
XLIII (May 1951), pp. 145–52; T. L.
Savitt, *Medicine and Slavery: The
Diseases and Health Care of Blacks
in Antebellum Virginia* (University
of Illinois Press, 1981); also, W.
Fisher, "The Use of Blacks for
Medical Experimentation and
Demonstration in the Old South,"
Journal of Southern History 48, no.
3 (1982), pp. 331–348; W. Weyers,
*The Abuse of Man: An Illustrated
History of Dubious Medical
Experimentation* (Ardor Scribendi,
2007); W. U. Eckart, *Medizin und
Kolonialimperialismus: Deutschland
1884–1945* (Paderborn: Schöningh,

1997); Jay Katz, Alexander Morgan
Capron (Author), Eleanor Swift
Glass (Author), *Experimentation
with Human Beings: The Authority
of the Investigator, Subject,
Professions, and State in the Human
Experimentation Process* (Russell
Sage Foundation, 1972).

106   reveals that African
Americans who had never heard
of the Tuskegee study: Dwayne
T. Brandon, Lydia A. Isaac, and
Thomas A. LaVeist, "The Legacy
of Tuskegee and Trust in Medical
Care: Is Tuskegee Responsible
for Race Differences in Mistrust
of Medical Care?" *Journal of the
National Medical Association* 97,
no. 7 (July, 2005), pp. 951–956.
Accessed at https://www.ncbi
.nlm.nih.gov/pmc/articles/PMC
2569322/.

106   reduced access to
healthcare in general and to
cardiac technology in particular:
Quinn Capers IV and Zarina
Sharalaya, "Racial Disparities in
Cardiovascular Care: A Review of
Culprits and Potential Solutions,"
*Journal of Racial and Ethnic Health
Disparities* 1 (2014), p. 171. Accessed
at https://link.springer.com/article
/10.1007/s40615-014-0021-7.

108   an online description of the
study by the university: Principal
Investigator: Samuel Tisherman,
MD, Professor of Surgery and
Director of the Division of Critical
Care and Trauma Education at the

University of Maryland School of Medicine, "Body Cooling Study." Accessed at https://www.umms .org/ummc/health-services /shock-trauma/news/body -cooling-study.

108 **"patients can withdraw from the study at any time":** Emergency Preservation and Resuscitation for Cardiac Arrest from Trauma (EPR-CAT. Accessed at https://www.umms.org/ummc /health-services/shock-trauma /news/body-cooling-study.

108 **According to a note on the study's online description:** Samuel Tisherman, "Body Cooling Study."

109 **medical-research results tend to emerge in concert with their commercial backers' financial interests:** Harriet A. Washington, "Flacking for Big Pharma: Drugmakers Don't Just Compromise Doctors; They Also Undermine the Top Medical Journals and Skew the Findings of Medical Research," *American Scholar*, Summer, 2011.

109 **Donna Haraway captures this when she writes:** Donna Haraway, "Situated Knowledges: The Science Question in Feminism and the Privilege of Partial Perspective," *Feminist Studies* 14, no. 3 (1988), pp. 575–599.

109 **there is also the ethical question of clinical equipoise:** B. Freedman, "Equipoise and the Ethics of Clinical Research," *New England Journal of Medicine* 317, no. 3 (1987), pp. 141–145; L. Shaw and T. Chalmers, "Ethics in Cooperative Clinical Trials," *Annals of the New York Academy of Sciences* 169 (1970), pp. 487–495.

110 **Baltimore was home to Henrietta Lacks:** Harriet A. Washington, "Limning the Semantics of Informed Consent," *American Journal of Law Medicine and Ethics*, September 1, 2016, p. X.

CHAPTER SIX

112 **He praised esketamine as a "stimulant":** Angela Chen, "The FDA Approved a New Ketamine Depression Drug—Here's What's Next," *The Verge,* March 11, 2019. Accessed at https://www.theverge .com/2019/3/11/18260297 /esketamine-fda-approval -depression-ketamine-clinic -science-health.

112 **esketamine, the "left-handed" form of the ketamine molecule:** "Esketamine Is the s-enantiomer [Left-Handed Mirror-Image Molecule] of Ketamine. Ketamine Is a Mixture of Two Enantiomers [Mirror-Image Molecules]." "FDA Approves New Nasal Spray Medication for Treatment-Resistant Depression; Available Only at a Certified Doctor's Office or Clinic," FDA press release, March 5, 2019.

184   Accessed at https://www.fda
.gov/news-events/press
-announcements/fda-approv.

**113   a lingering disruption
of attention, learning, and
memory:** Public Citizen, et al,
"Letter to Scott Gottlieb, FDA
Commissioner, RE: Prospective
Clinical Trials Comparing the
Safety and Effectiveness of
Ketamine with Those of Other
Drugs for Management of Agitation
Were Conducted Without the
Informed Consent of the Subjects,
in Violation of Federal Human
Subjects Protection Regulations,"
Letter to FDA and OHRP Regarding
Prospective Clinical Trials Testing
Ketamine for Agitation, July 25,
2018. Accessed at https://
www.citizen.org/wp-content
/uploads/2442.pdf.

**113   better known by its
subterranean alter ego:**
"Commonly Abused Drugs Charts,"
National Institute on Drug Abuse,
Revised July 2019. Accessed at
https://www.drugabuse.gov/drugs
-abuse/commonly-abused-drugs
-charts.

**113   "there are no FDA-approved
medications to treat addiction to
ketamine":** "Commonly Abused
Drugs Charts," National Institute
on Drug Abuse.

**113   six people who had been
administered the drug died:** Peter
Cary, "Trump's Praise Put Drug
for Vets on Fast Track, but Experts

Aren't Sure It Works," The Center
for Public Integrity, June 18, 2019.
Accessed at https://publicintegrity
.org/politics/trumps-raves-put
-drug-for-vets-on-fast-track-but
-experts-arent-sure-it-works/.

**113   unimpressed enough to vote
against including esketamine:**
Peter Cary, "Controversial J & J
Drug Pushed by Trump Nixed from
VA's Pharmacy List," The Center
for Public Integrity, June 21, 2019.
Accessed at https://publicintegrity
.org/federal-politics/controversial
-anti-depression-drug-pushed-by
-president-trump-is-nixed-from
-vas-pharmacy-list/.

**114   Trump subsequently
touted Spravato's "incredible"
effectiveness:** Peter Cary,
"Controversial J & J Drug Pushed
by Trump Nixed from VA's
Pharmacy List."

**114   the FDA did approve
Spravato:** Jon Hamilton, "FDA
Approves Esketamine Nasal Spray
For Hard-to-Treat Depression,"
NPR, March 5, 2019. Accessed at
https://www.npr.org/sections
/health-shots/2019/03/05
/700509903/fda-clears
-esketamine-nasal-spray-for
-hard-to-treat-depression.

**114   the FDA appears to
inappropriately discount the
possibility:** Peter Cary, "Trump's
Praise Put Drug for Vets on Fast
Track, but Experts Aren't Sure It
Works."

114 **unless drugs can be shown to kill patients outright:** Peter Lurie, MD, MPH, and Sidney M. Wolfe, MD, "FDA Medical Officers Report Lower Standards Permit Dangerous Drug Approvals," Public Citizen, December 2, 1998. Accessed at http://www.citizen.org/hrg1466; Wolfe, "Congressional Testimony on FDA Deficiencies." Cited in Harriet A. Washington, *Deadly Monopolies*, p. 140.

114 **"Everything is approvable":** Peter Lurie, MD, MPH, and Sidney M. Wolfe, MD, "FDA Medical Officers Report Lower Standards Permit Dangerous Drug Approvals," p. 140.

115 **New York State had amassed 82,000 DNA profiles:** Edgar Sandoval "N.Y.P.D. to Remove DNA Profiles of Non-Criminals from Database," *New York Times,* February 20, 2020.

116 **Ketamine Administration from "MPD Involvement in Pre-Hospital Sedation Final Report":** "MPD Involvement in Pre-Hospital Sedation Final Report," Minneapolis Office of Police Conduct Review, July 16, 2018, p. 10. Accessed at https://lims .minneapolismn.gov/Download /File/1389/Office percent20of percent20Police percent20Conduct percent20Review percent20(OPCR) percent20PreHosptial percent20 Sedation percent20Study percent20 Final percent20Report.pdf.

117 **On December 16, 2017, Brittany Buckley:** Brittany J. Buckley, Plaintiff, vs. Hennepin County; Hennepin Healthcare System, Inc.; Hennepin Healthcare Research Institute; Paramedics Anthony D'Agostino, Katherine A. Kaufmann, and Jonathan R. Thomalia, all in their individual and official capacities; William Heegaard, MD, Jon Cole, MD, Jeffrey Ho, MD, Paul Nystrom, MD, Craig Peine, MD, Karen Heim-Duthoy, PharmD, and Researches J. Does 1–10, whose identities are presently unknown to Plaintiff, all in their individual and official capacities, Case 0:18-cv-03124-JNE-DTS, Document 1, Filed 11/07/18, Page 13 of 22, Footnote 37.

119 **denies that Brittany met the study criteria:** Andy Mannix, "Patients Sedated by Ketamine Were Enrolled in Hennepin Healthcare Study," *Minneapolis Star Tribune,* June 23, 2018. Accessed at http://www.startribune.com /patients-sedated-by-ketamine -were-enrolled-in-hennepin -healthcare-study/486363071/.

119 **As Brittany watched them prepare the injection:** "As defendant Paramedics Anthony D'Agostino, Katherine A. Kaufmann, and Jonathan R. Thomalia drew up medication in a syringe, Ms. Buckley saw that she was about to be injected with an unknown medication and verbally objected." Case 0:18-cv-03124

186   -JNE-DTS, Document 1, Filed 11/07/18, Page 13. Footnote 37.

121   **being forced to participate in medical research has been permitted:** "CFR—Code of Federal Regulations Title 21." Accessed at https://www .accessdata.fda.gov/scripts /cdrh/cfdocs/cfcfr/CFRsearch .cfm?CFRPart=50.

121   **researchers used yet another end run around consent:** "Clinical Trial Informed Consent Form Posting (45 CFR 46.116(h))," U.S. Department of Health and Human Services Office for Human Research Protections. Accessed at https:// www.hhs.gov/ohrp/regulations -and-policy/informed-consent -posting/index.html; and "Informed Consent Requirements in Emergency Research (OPRR Letter, 1996)." Accessed at https://www.hhs.gov/ohrp /regulations-and-policy/guidance /emergency-research-informed -consent-requirements/index .html; https://www.hhs.gov/ohrp /regulations-and-policy/informed -consent-posting/index.html.

121   **with a document that had been left for her to sign:** Complaint, CASE 0:18-cv-03124 -JNE-DTS, Document 1, Filed 11/07/18, Page 12 of 22, 13.

122   **federal judge dismissed Brittany's lawsuit:** Andy Mannix,

"Judge Throws Out Patient's Ketamine Lawsuit Against HCMC: Woman Says That Hennepin Healthcare Violated Her Civil Rights," *Minneapolis Star Tribune*, September 16, 2019. Accessed at http://www.startribune.com /andy-mannix/366674391.

122   **ketamine experiments involving dozens of people sedated by paramedics:** Andy Mannix, "Ketamine Probe Will Examine Conduct of Officers," *Minneapolis Star-Tribune*, June 21, 2018. Accessed at http://www .startribune.com/ketamine -probe-will-examine-conduct -of-officers/486207731/.

123   **a Level-I trauma center:** "Trauma Center Designations and Levels," American Trauma Society, January 1, 2000. Accessed at https://braintrauma .org/news/article/trauma-center -designations.

124   **urged an investigation into the conduct of the clinical trials:** Michael Carome, MD, "Unethical Human Experiments That Tested Powerful General Anesthetic for Agitation," *Health Letter,* September 2018. Accessed at https://www .citizen.org/news/outrage-of -the-month-unethical-human -experimentation-in-2015 -and-our-broken-system-for -protecting-human-research -subjects/.

CHAPTER SEVEN

126 **What would a typical physician say about this research study?:** Parth Shah, Imani Thornton, Danielle Turrin, and John E. Hipskind, "Informed Consent" (updated August 22, 2020), StatPearls Publishing, January 2020. Accessed at https://www.ncbi.nlm.nih.gov/books/NBK430827/.

126 **The responsibility to communicate this information persists throughout the study:** "Inside Clinical Trials: Testing Medical Products in People," U.S. Food And Drug Administration, November 6, 2014. Accessed at https://www.fda.gov/Drugs/Drug-Information-Consumers/Inside-Clinical-Trials-Testing-Medical-Products-People Consumers/Inside-Clinical-Trials-Testing-Medical-Products-People; Last Accessed March 7, 2020.

127 **informed consent is required for treatment:** "Inside Clinical Trials: Testing Medical Products in People," U.S. Food And Drug Administration.

129 **conflicts of interest rife in the medical industry extend to some ethicists:** Harriet A. Washington, "Limning The Semantic Frontier of Informed Consent," *Journal Of Law, Medicine & Ethics* 44 (2016), pp. 381–393.

130 **1996 addenda to the Code of Federal Regulations:** "Minutes, September 4, 2018, 6:00–8:00 p.m.," Ethics & Medical-Legal Affairs Committee, John Murphy Conference Room.

130 **medical and policy experts concerned with clinical trial safety:** Barry Meier, "An Overseer of Medical Trials Comes Under Fire," *New York Times*, March 26, 2009. Accessed at https://www.nytimes.com/2009/03/27/business/27clinic.html.

131 **Coast directly or indirectly reviewed studies:** Alicia Mundy, "Coast IRB, Caught in Sting, to Close," *Wall Street Journal*, April 22, 2009. Accessed at https://www.wsj.com/articles/SB124042341694744375.

132 **the GAO sprinkled ample clues throughout the proposal:** Alicia Mundy, "Lawmakers Detail Medical Research Sting: Company Was a Real Dog," *Wall Street Journal*, March 26, 2009. Note that this account misspells the name of the product. It's correct spelling is "Adhesiabloc."

132 **rejected it outright, dismissing the trial as "awful" and "a piece of junk":** Barry Meier, "An Overseer of Medical Trials Comes Under Fire."

132 **However, Coast approved it:** Nancy Walton, "An Update on

188   the Coast IRB Sting," *Research Ethics Blog*. Accessed at https://researchethicsblog.com.

133   **questioning the government sting's legality and ethics:** "Congressional 'Sting' Operation Uncovered," Applied Clinical Trials Editors, press release, March 12, 2009. Accessed at http://www.appliedclinicaltrialsonline.com/congressional-sting-operation-uncovered.

133   **"I cannot believe that my government did this to me and my company":** Barry Meier, "An Overseer of Medical Trials Comes Under Fire."

133   **A number of Coast's "key customers" then defected:** Nick Taylor, "Coast IRB Closes Doors After GAO Sting," Outsourcing-Pharma.com, April 26, 2009. Accessed at https://www.outsourcing-pharma.com/Article/2009/04/27/Coast-IRB-closes-doors-after-GAO sting?Utm_source=copyright&utm_medium=onsite&utm_campaign=copyright.

136   **did not always go smoothly:** Lila Guterman, "Guinea Pigs in the ER," *Chronicle of Higher Education* 52, no. 41 (June 16, 2006), pp. A14–A18.

136   **enrolling 22,000 unwitting subjects:** Rob Stein, "Critical Care Without Consent; Ethicists Disagree on Experimenting During Crises," *Washington Post*, May 27, 2007, p. A01.

137   **you cannot predict when someone will suffer cardiac arrest:** Sudden cardiac arrest ensues when the coordinated electrical signals that generate an orderly, regular heartbeat become deranged, fall into arrhythmia, and the heart suddenly stops, a victim of ventricular fibrillation electrical malfunction.

138   **70 percent said they had no objection to that trial:** Lila Guterman, "Guinea Pigs in the ER."

139   **Use of the device cost twenty people their lives:** Marcus Eng Hock Ong, Joseph P. Ornato, David P. Edwards, et al, "Use of an Automated, Load-Distributing Band Chest Compression Device for Out-of-Hospital Cardiac Arrest Resuscitation," *JAMA* 295, no. 22 (2006), pp. 2629–2637. doi: 10.1001/jama.295.22.2629.

139   **the very first study to utilize the 50.23 loophole:** Thomas Ming Swi Chang, "Strategies for New Generations of HBOCs," *Artificial Cells, Blood Substitutes, and Biotechnology* 38, no. 6 (2010). Accessed at https://www.tandfonline.com/doi/full/10.3109/10731199.2010.526365.

140   **the study had to be stopped when these subjects died:** One study author, Charles Nathanson, later noted that he stood to profit from his research findings because he had developed a method of decreasing problems created by

the blood substitutes. He didn't disclose this conflict of interest, but frankly, the printed disclosure of such conflicts that many journals require is a poor substitute for refusing to publish work that has been tainted by financial bias.

141 **essentially no one knew anything about the trial or the substance:** Glenn McGee, PhD, "The Wonders of Polyheme ... By Press Release," Bioethics.net, January 9, 2009. Accessed at http://www.bioethics.net/2009/01/the-wonders-of-polyhemeby-press-release/.

142 **which he acknowledged was only a "tiny fraction":** during a March 17 radio interview.

CONCLUSION

148 **favored the sponsoring company's experimental heart drugs and often its devices:** Harriet A. Washington, "Flacking for Big Pharma."

150 **the science-challenged Trump administration banned seven terms from official use:** Lena H. Sun and Juliet Eilperin, "CDC Gets List of Forbidden Words: Fetus, Transgender, Diversity," *Washington Post*, December 15, 2017.

150 **The overall intent of this latter-day newspeak is clear:** George Orwell, "Appendix: The Principles of Newspeak."

152 **more semantic manipulations of research subjects have been used to bar their consent:** Harriet A. Washington, "Limning the Semantic Frontier of Informed Consent."

153 **Since 2006, I have suggested integral changes to IRB composition:** Harriet A. Washington, *Medical Apartheid*, p. 401.

156 **Such lapses would be discouraged by the adoption of a "devil's advocate" strategy:** Robert J. Joustra, "The Tenth Man," *Capital Commentary*, November 1, 2013. Accessed at https://www.cpjustice.org/public/capital_commentary/article/264. "Following the recommendation of the Agranat Commission in 1973–1974, Military Intelligence established a Control Unit that was expected to play this role of the devil's advocate. Its responsibility was to produce a range of explanations and assessments of events that avoided relying on a single concept, as happened in 1973. Brooks puts it a bit more dramatically: If ten people are in a room, and nine agree on how to interpret and respond to a situation, the tenth man must disagree. His duty is to find the best possible argument for why the decision of the group is flawed."

Columbia Global Reports is a publishing imprint from Columbia University that commissions authors to do original on-site reporting around the globe on a wide range of issues. The resulting novella-length books offer new ways to look at and understand the world that can be read in a few hours. Most readers are curious and busy. Our books are for them.

Subscribe to Columbia Global Reports and get six books a year in the mail in advance of publication. globalreports.columbia.edu/subscribe

The Call: Inside the Global Saudi Religious Project
Krithika Varagur

The Socialist Awakening: What's Different Now About The Left
John B. Judis

Ghosting the News: Local Journalism and the Crisis of American Democracy
Margaret Sullivan

The Agenda : How a Republican Supreme Court Is Reshaping America
Ian Millhiser

Reading Our Minds: The Rise of Big Data Psychiatry
Daniel Barron

Freedomville: The Story of a 21st-Century Slave Revolt
Laura T. Murphy